OUT OF THE DARKNESS:
Coping With Disability

by Robert Lovering

ISBN #0-9615213-0-8

Phoenix, Arizona

Published by:
Associated Rehabilitation Counseling Specialists (ARCS) 1993

Outline — Table of Contents

About The Title iv

Getting Into The Mood viii

1 Newly Diagnosed

- What? Not Me! 1
- Denial 3
- Fantasy 5
- Reality 7
- Depression 8
- Bitterness/Anger 11
- Fear 12
- Challenges 14
- Sources Of Help 16
- A New Sense Of Direction 19

2 Parents Of Handicapped Children

- Thunderstorms Of Life 21
- Beating The Odds 24
- Fight Or Surrender 26
- It's Okay To Cry 29
- I'm Not Courageous—I'm Frightened 32
- You Can't Do It Alone 34
- I'll Give My Life 36
- There Must Be Something I Can Do 38
- Looking From Inside Out 40

3 Family And Friends

- Hands-on Care By Spouse Or Family Member 44
- Money! Money! Money! 46
- Home Sweet Home 47
- Frayed Emotions 51
- Oh, For The Crystal Ball 53
- For Mother, Father, Sisters And Brothers 53
- For Friends And Relatives 57

4 Disabled And The World

- Attitudes Make The Difference 63
- Celebrating A Disability 72
- Well, What Else Can We Do? 74
- Doctors, Hospitals, And Medical Practitioners 78

5 REMOVING LIMITS TO OUR INDEPENDENCE

Architectural Barriers 82
Possible Solutions And Alternatives 84
Bathrooms 86
Kitchens 88
Floor Covering 89
Environmental Barriers 91

6 MANAGING STRESS AND ANGER

What Is Stress? 93
Can We Always Recognize Stress? 95
What Damage Can Stress Do To Our Bodies? 96
Is Stress Additive? 97
What About Pain? 98
How Can We Control Our Anger? 99

7 MARRIED COUPLES

The Stress Of Disability in Marriage 102
Flexibility In Marriage 103
Hard-Hat Areas In Marriage 105
Does Disability Mean Divorce? 108

8 TOOLS FOR EMOTIONAL COPING

Developing Your Tools 114
Parallels In Coping With Stress 116
Get Life Into Prospective 117
Use Diversional Tactics 119
Occupy Your Mind 119

9 SUICIDE CONCERNS

Relationship Of Suicide And Depression 121
How Common Is Suicide? 122
Why Do People Take Their Own Lives? 123
How Are Suicide And Disability Related? 124
Are There Any Absolutes? 126

10 RELIGION, THE TABOO SUBJECT

What's Important About Religion? 128
Back To Basics 130
Faith And Disability 133
The Crutch Of Faith 135

About The Title

When we say *coping,* what do we mean? In wood working a common tool is a coping saw. It is so named because it is capable of making intricate curves in fitting pieces of wood together, or one piece coping or fitting with the other.

Coping in general means: "Struggling or contending with on fairly even terms or with some degree of success." Synonyms are encounter, struggle, compete, contend, strive, engage, face, confront, hold one's own, manage, hold at bay, combat on equal terms.

That is what this book is all about. It is to help you manage or contend with living life as a person with a disability. And I might as well get it off my chest now at the very beginning. I am sick and tired of this so-called political correctness garbage. I am tired of those who wear their feelings on their sleeves hoping someone will make some sort of ethnic, minority group, gender, political, or whatever statement over which they can take righteous offense. If you are one of those people, kindly do me a favor and stop reading, toss this in a waste container, or just pass this book on to someone else who is not wearing his feelings on his sleeve. Do yourself and me a favor by not bothering to write or call me and inform me of my offense.

A rose by any other name is still a rose; manure by any other name still has the same stench; and so does the asinine new politically-correct word, *physically challenged,* or any of the other new names for those of us with physical disabilities. What an absolute misnomer. When any of the professional basketball teams come out onto the floor, *they* are physically challenged, but they certainly are not disabled in any sense of the word. Using a so-called positive word to describe a negative situation never has and never will change the situation.

There came across my desk a delightful article copied from the *St. Paul Pioneer Press*, St. Paul, Minnesota, dated 11/23/92. My original intention was to quote a few lines from it for you and then go on. Unfortunately it is too good for that, so here it is in its entirety.

Reprinted by Permission

Viewpoint

Constant changes in 'correct' labels wears down disabled man's patience

by **DR. MARVIN THOMPSON**, GUEST COLUMNIST

As everyone knows, there is a good deal of argument taking place on various university campuses concerning "political correctness." The controversy is noisy for everyone, but very personal because it involves what I am supposed to be called—"disabled" or whatever.

I had polio when I was 10 and since then I have been in a wheelchair. I am now retired, a professor emeritus of St. Cloud State University.

In 1933 I was in an iron lung for three weeks at the University of Minnesota Hospitals in the wing for crippled children. And for 18 months after that I was at Gillette State Hospital for Crippled Children.

Later I lived with my parents in Minneapolis, but I was taken by bus each day to Dowling School for Crippled Children. Then to Marshall High where along with other handicapped students I attended regular classes.

During four years at Macalester College and six years of graduate work at the University of Minnesota, I may have been regarded as handicapped or as disabled. No one bothered to tell me and I didn't ask. In 1952 I taught high school for one year at the Crippled Children's School in Jamestown, N.D. (since renamed The Anne Carlson School).

Finally I came to St. Cloud State where I was on the faculty from 1956 until I retired in 1980. These were very happy years, with fine faculty and students, during which I taught Shakespeare and was regarded, I think, as a good teacher. For official purposes I was considered by the administration as disabled, I suppose, but it didn't seem to matter to my students or to me.

But sometime in the 1980's, all hell broke loose across the country in the academic naming game. To my amazement I found that during my lifetime I had not been crippled or handicapped at all, or even disabled. No, during all that time without my knowing it, I had been *otherly abled.*

Right? Wrong! Because before I had a chance retroactively to get used to that new term, they had already changed it to *physically challenged.* Right? No, wrong again. *Differently abled* was what I now had been, and if you don't agree with that terminology, you are guilty of *ableism.*

It may sound funny, but if you happen to teach at a university today, it's no joke. It means that if you don't use the most up-to-date, politically correct language, you can be legally in trouble on matters of retention, tenure, and promotion.

But even though I am retired now and beyond the reach of the politically-correct crowd, I still would like to ask someone just what kind of lunacy is going on here and who is responsible for it.

I would guess that if it's anyone, it's the human relations and/or various special studies departments. I also think that the whole thing is not so much liberal or conservative as it is crypto-fascist.

To whomever it applies, may I say that I am still in a wheelchair as I have been for 60 years, and that I studied and worked hard in order to teach Shakespeare and publish and contribute to the discipline of English.

And I'll be damned if I'll let some self-appointed expert from outside any discipline at all tell me how I should define my physical condition. This is my life and it's my business how I choose to describe myself.

Oh, and one more bit of retroactive insanity. Because I am seated in a wheelchair and necessarily have to look up at other people when I talk with them, I have also been *vertically challenged* all this time, would you believe?

Now look: After a good life my polio body is tiring—as is true with many in this country who are suffering the fatigue of post-polio syndrome. But if anybody tries to use phony PC language to me, I promise to rise up out of my wheelchair like the Ghost of Crippled Past and hit him or her in the mouth.

Enough is enough.

★ ★ ★

Now it would appear to me that the politically-correct crowd has lost its prospective, or it never had one. To me these PC persons are characteristic of the old axiom: "An empty wagon makes the most noise." So many of these self-appointed "officers of the day" are all bark and no bite (noise without substance). They carry protest signs and shout slogans, and then return home thinking they have really done their civic and moral duty. Personally, I am sick unto death of protests, slogans, marches, et al. If you want to change the world, do something constructive—change yourself first, be a good example and perhaps others might follow. Carrying signs of protest and shouting slogans (usually sprinkled with expletives) just turns me OFF.

If the word handicapped or disabled offends you when no offense is intended, *you* indeed have a problem. A word can only transmit offense when offense is intended. Your attitude may offend me, but not your terms. If you want to get technical if not politically correct, I am a cripple— C-R-I-P-P-L-E. Does that offend you? No, it does not offend me. The dictionary defines a cripple as anyone who has lost the *functional* use of any of his extremities. Personally, first and foremost I am a person; second and insignificantly, one with a physical disability.

Let's spend our time working out the problems of life rather than fussing about what we or anyone else is called. Let's work on removing architectural barriers, employment barriers, transportation barriers, and prejudice based on myths and half-truths. Let's focus our attention beyond gender, race, ethnicity, physical size or shape. When you shake my hand, look me in the face and not let your mind or your eyes wander to my wheelchair. It is only a means of mobility!

As long as I am on my soapbox, I might as well finish with another gripe. In *OUT OF THE ORDINARY: A Digest on Disability,* it was strongly suggested that I change several words so that some people would not be offended. In one instance I used the term snotty (and the word was a perfect fit), but was changed to arrogant. This time around I am not cow-towing to any group or person. There will be no changing to make this book palatable. There will be no sugar coating. It will be printed as it was conceived. If others are allowed to censor what is written in this book, you would receive 100+ blank pages.

GETTING INTO THE MOOD

If this had been titled Preface, most likely many of you would have overlooked it. In my years as a high school student, one of the things I never did was to read the preface of any book. My mind just wanted to get into it and get going. It was not until many years later that it finally dawned upon me how important those few paragraphs were to set the scene and give reading some direction. Who was writing the book? What was the purpose of the author? To whom was the book targeted?

Who in the world cares about the author's age, experience in certain backgrounds or disciplines, education, etc. If you want to understand the book you first must understand the author. Did we not learn that in Literature 101? So if you did not read "About The Author" on the back cover, do it now before you read another word.

Who is writing this book? Well, he is now gray, balding, and plumpish (notice I did not say fat), 6'0'' in height, who spends 100% of his waking hours in a wheelchair. And he is a white, anglo-saxon Protestant who has spent his entire adult life grubbing out facts on disability. At first they were grubbed to solve his own problems; later these facts were gathered to help solve the problems of others. Did he choose this profession? No, it chose him.

If there had been anything else that he could do and not feel guilty, he would have done it. However, he would have been overcome by guilt having answers to so many problems facing persons with disabilities and turning his back on those in need. If not a counselor to persons with disabilities, into what vocation would he have entered? Perhaps it would have been mechanical or electrical engineering. He grew up in the printing trades so perhaps it might have been printing.

These pages are coming to you because I want you to be able to benefit from my education and experience. You most likely will not agree with some of my advice. You may dislike my philosophy of life and my philosophy of disability. That is your privilege, but at least you have it before you to ponder. The book is simple, not profound!

With a subject as broad as disability, one would expect this book to be a potpourri of topics—and it is. Perhaps it would be interesting for you to know how each chapter came into being.

Chapter 1 for the Newly Diagnosed was born out of a request by the Southwest Desert Chapter of the National Multiple Sclerosis Society. There was a lack of down-to-earth, sensible reading material for those who had just been diagnosed. Would I write something for them?

Chapter 2 for Parents of Handicapped Children also came about from a request from the director of United Cerebral Palsy of West Central Wisconsin, and for the same reason: "We need practical information that our parents can understand and use."

Chapter 3 for Family and Friends was the result of a query by Frank Billingsley, a board member of a local group seeking to establish a residential facility for persons who were severely disabled. A friend of his suffered a stroke and the family was totally lost in this maze of treatment and rehabilitation. "Do you have anything for them?" he asked. No, but something could be written.

Chapter 4 for the Disabled and the World, and Chapter 5 on Removing Limits to our Independence had no specific stimulant other than the vital importance I had seen in these areas over the years.

Chapters 6, 7, and 8 on Stress/Anger, Marriage, and Emotional Coping are the current buzz words in the socio/psychological world of counseling. The book would be "missing a tooth" without them.

Chapter 9 on Suicide Concerns became a viable topic during the writing and editing of this book because a young mother took her life—blind from birth, with two small children, and recently disabled in an collision with an automobile. We spent many hours together in an attempt to sort out her feelings. Her final statement to me was, "I can cope with blindness, but not blindness *and* being *crippled.*" Her suicide and all concerns that went with it was very fresh in my mind.

Chapter 10 on Religion began as a six-page booklet designed to be left with those who were referred to us by our local health agencies. Care had to be taken not to offend or anger any of those who were referred. It was hand-given or left on a table with the statement, "I want you to know this is religious in nature. I think it is very important. If you are not interested simply throw it away." However, it was discovered that when our literature was displayed at seminars, health fairs and conventions, this booklet was gobbled up in astounding numbers.

It would be my hope that you would not find any mechanical or other errors in this text., but you will. Please know that every possible method was used to eliminate errors, but they always seem to creep in to embarrass the author.

There are times when the words he/himself are left to stand rather than the he/she, himself/herself busines. And sometimes in similar instances I have chosen to use they/them or themselves in place of the correct use of the singular.

My use of the first person singular may bother some of you. It would be more literally correct to use the third person or use such terms as *the author*. However, the first person is purposely used because I covet for the two of us—the reader and the writer—the closeness and intimacy of a face-to-face conversation.

I have not taken space to tell some of my usual jokes or stories—and I am a joke teller. There have been many humorous incidents in my life relating to disability, but you won't find them in these pages. This book is serious stuff.

Bob

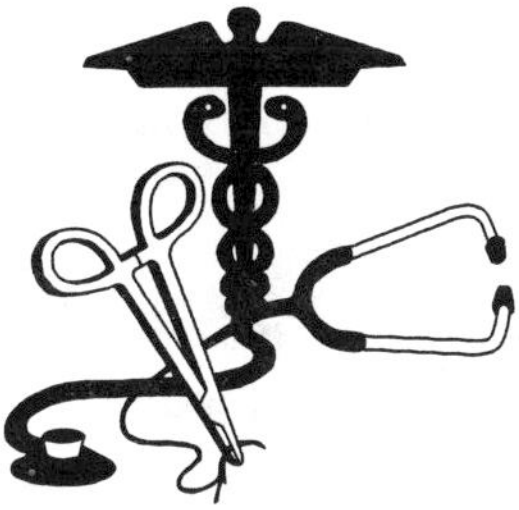

Chapter 1

THE NEWLY DIAGNOSED

WHAT? NOT ME!

Recently you were confronted by a circumstance that will no doubt in time be considered the greatest challenge of your life—a diagnosis of a potentially-disabling disease or condition, or a struggle with a life-threatening illness. This diagnosis has or will affect every aspect of your life. The following quote from a person high in the corporate structure may help you grasp that sense of suddenly being lost in darkness and not knowing which way to turn:

> "To me my first morning was the feeling of a typical person newly diagnosed as having MS, having the feeling that nothing you have or have learned will help you on your way to—you know not where. The person newly diagnosed is so hurt, confused, and concerned that he cannot function.
>
> My first question was WHAT? That was quickly replaced with, NOT ME! What will I do? Did they really tell me the truth? Pity, pity for Mike. Do I tell or not tell? Oh, my job, my family, my everything. Cry all night, but now it is morning, the first day of the rest of my life and I don't know what to do.
>
> For the first time I really don't know or have any idea of what to do. I don't even know anyone to see, to call, or anything, and it is still morning of the first day. What do I do?"

The purpose of this chapter is to assist in this challenge by drawing from my experience as a professional counselor in the field of disability, and as one who has been personally challenged by a disability for over forty-seven years. My answers may not be your answers, nor my ways your ways. Nonetheless, it is an opportunity to share with you those facts and feelings that may contribute to greater understanding of your future.

First of all, does our "diagnosis" make us different from other persons or does it make us different from what we were prior to this new challenge? Did my bout with polio forty-something years ago and my life in a wheelchair since then change me as a person? Of course it changed my mobility and limited many of my choices. It changed the direction of my life and it gave me unique experiences. However, I am the same person. Do not allow yourself to fall into the trap of seeing yourself as now being basically different from other members of society. Although I must roll down the sidewalk, apart from my mode of mobility I am no different from those walkers whom I pass or who pass by me. Am I a disabled person? No, I am a person *first,* with a disability *second*—a person with a disability. There is a difference!

Obviously there are some limitations placed upon us by the dictates of our diagnosis, but our expectations from society should be to be treated just like everyone else—because we are just like everyone else. However, we do appreciate understanding and consideration regarding those limits that have been placed upon us by our disease or condition. Society does not "owe" us anything because we have our limitations. Avoid the we/they syndrome: we, the disabled or limited, and they—those who are not. This type of thinking only leads to hostilities and war—we against them. And you know that everyone loses in war.

One of the universal problems you all will face is how to tactfully handle those well-meaning family members and friends who insist upon calling you or mailing every newspaper article they feel is related to your situation, or continuously asking about your health. Even strangers have approached me on the street to tell me of some treatment or clinic that they thought might help me, or that if I would pray or believe a certain way I would be made whole. Not even your anger or rudeness will stifle these well-meaning persons. They have a cause and a calling that they must fulfill. You cannot change them, but you can change yourself. Don't waste your time being hurt or angry. Just accept their good intentions, smile, and thank them—friends, and strangers alike. You may be more direct with close family members. Tell them how you feel, but it is my opinion that there is never an excuse for rudeness—never.

There are also a series of emotional stages that have come to be associated with loss—any disaster or trauma. Many years before I had heard of any of these, my experience with myself and others told me that there were emotional steps to recovery. It seemed to be a process that was not absolute, but that generally followed a pattern. Some avoided a stage altogether, and some became hung up on one for life.

Denial

The first step after a devastating diagnosis was denial. There was a mistake in diagnosis; we do not have this disease or condition. Some of us told ourselves that the diagnosis was no doubt correct, but somehow we were going to beat the odds even if they might be a million to one. Others of us were convinced that somehow God would look down favorably upon us and miraculously heal us, thus beating the odds. After all, we were not such bad people, and that when we attracted God's attention he would realize the error.

In retrospect, my own denial seemed to be in short steps. Even though all the symptoms were present, until the spinal tap found live polio virus in my spinal fluid, my mind told me that there had to be a mistake somewhere. I would be okay again. Other times this denial was manifest in day dreaming telling myself that this—all of it—was just a dream and that in the morning it would all be gone and my life would continue as it had been: walking, running, working, going to school, etc.

Some have told me that they never experienced denial, and that may be true for a few. But the great majority of us had a period of denial that may have lasted from a few seconds to many years, even for a lifetime. Sometimes the greatest denial of all is that of denying denial.

Regardless, if persons deny they have a problem of any kind or degree, there can be no solution. There can be no activity toward solving or accepting the reality of a problem that "does not exist." My guess is that the fact you are reading this indicates that it is unlikely you are denying (in denial of) the problem of a diagnosis to yourself or someone you care about deeply.

Those who have had considerable medical experience such as doctors, nurses, and other health professionals tend to have shorter terms of denial. After all, they do not possess the naiveté as those of us who are not so well experienced and informed. We must understand denial from the standpoint of emotional survival just as we understand any survival behavior—even instances of cannibalism such as in the Donner Party.

When our emotions are so devastated that we are on the verge of a total emotional breakdown and other defense mechanisms have failed to disrupt the shattering process, the weapon of last resort is denial. This should help us to understand that denial is a normal response to emotional survival. Persons who are in denial are simply trying to tell the world that they have reached the last straw, and that they cannot at this moment tolerate reality.

What the family, spouse, friends, and those of us who are professional counselors must understand is the potential danger in attempting to rush an emotionally-traumatized person into reality before one is emotionally ready. So often we attempt to "drive" the person out of denial, and it can be devastating rather than helpful. It is my opinion that when a person has emotionally healed to the point of accepting the reality of the diagnosis, the move from denial to reality will generally be automatic and self effected.

How about those persons who continue on and on in denial far beyond what we believe to be comparable with the devastation? Keep in mind that each of us is an individual; therefore, there is no rule that should indicate when we should have our eyes opened. Many of those with whom my experience lies in long-term denial simply were not ready and could not open their eyes to reality without total emotional breakdown and emotional disintegration. Therefore, in my counseling practice it has not been my goal to drive persons from denial, but rather to help them begin the orderly process of emotional healing. Emotional healing takes time just as does physical healing, some persons and some injuries take longer than others.

We also must understand that healing, be it physical or emotional healing, is not instantaneous. From the early moments of denial of the doctor's diagnosis of polio to the time when my mind could accept the reality that there was not going to be a miraculous healing or even normal physical improvement, I was dancing on the step of denial. It was a slow process that extended nearly nine months before true reality set in.

Fantasy

Although it might appear that my mind was in a serious state of denial nine months, it was really only for about four months. The remaining five months were more in the vein of fantasy. Fantasy seems to be the last vestige of denial, but it is part of the emotional survival mechanism and therefore it is normal.

It was common for the group of ten men in our polio ward to dream of some crazy scheme to be whole again. One time it came to me as a delightful and pleasant thought that perhaps I might fall out of bed and strike a key nerve in my body that would restore my paralyzed legs and trunk. In those days "Invisible Scarlet O'Neal" appeared in the comic strips. She could press a nerve on her wrist and become invisible; perhaps I could find a nerve to press to make me walk.

Couldn't there be some unknown treatment somewhere that would restore us? How about a specific diet, a certain doctor or prescription? The fantasy step of disability makes us vulnerable to "quack" doctors, treatments, and remedies. My parents heard of a clinic in South Dakota that had reported miraculous healings: the blind saw, and the cripples walked. Could they live with themselves if they did not do all in their power to get me there? They did—no miracle. I came home in the same wheelchair and one step closer to reality.

Much of my Phoenix practice has been with those with multiple sclerosis. Every new idea that comes along captures a few. They travel to Mexico or Europe to some clinic reported to cure, stabilize, or greatly improve their symptoms. They try this diet or that, or overdose on megavitamins. Some have all their teeth fillings replaced with gold (or in some cases the teeth extracted) because they have heard that the mercury in tooth fillings is the cause of their ills. Some rid themselves of their dogs and cats because it was reported that they may be a cause. Others have been injected with snake venom (seriously). Don't laugh! There is no limit to what any of us will do in our quest for an improvement or a cure. However, most of our attempts end in failure.

Fantasy, as is denial, is a necessary ingredient in coping with the early emotional throes caused by disability. Jill Kinmont, in the biographical movie of her skiing accident, "The Other Side of the

Mountain," gritted her teeth and said emphatically, "I am going to walk out of here if it is the last thing I do." Most of us who are disabled have said this or some other self-promise to "beat" our disability, and we meant it; but it was a hope—a fantasy, defined in the dictionary as "a supposition based on no solid foundation"—a hope we needed to endure the moment.

As I watched the movie and heard those determined words, a lump grew in my throat. Thirty years earlier I had said the same thing, with the same determination, and also with the same results—a lifetime of paralysis. My emotional reaction to those words surprised me. Hadn't this been buried many years ago?

Keep in mind that fantasy is not unhealthy. It is in the makeup of all healthy persons. We daydream—we fulfill our wishes and destroy our enemies in our imaginations. If we see ourselves as ugly, we imagine ourselves as ravishingly beautiful. We embody ourselves in the Charles Atlas ads to rescue us from being the "97-pound weakling." Fantasy entertains children and fantasy fulfills psychological needs in adults. The danger lies in not recognizing the fact of fantasy—when we begin to accept the figments of our fantasies as facts. As long as we recognize fantasy as fiction, and as long as we are its master and not its slave, it is a wonderful aspirin for the pain of reality.

One person in my experience stands out as an excellent example of a detrimental fantasy having a happy ending. It is taken directly from *OUT OF THE ORDINARY: A Digest on Disability.*

> "Many persons with a disability, even with poorer odds, live a day-to-day existence with a hope—a destructive hope—that tomorrow a miracle will transform them into wholeness.
>
> "Miller is not a Spanish surname, but when I responded to the referral from the Visiting Nurse Service, I found Joe to be very Hispanic and very disabled from multiple sclerosis. His nurse told me he was not interested in any treatment or long-range planning because he felt he was not going to need treatment and lessons on self help. He had absolute faith; Jesus was going to heal him. He just sat there day after day waiting for the miracle.
>
> "Each day, as he had for many months, he sent his son down the street to the flower shop to buy a rose to replace that one purchased yesterday—one that he had given to Jesus and that had wilted. His faith remained steadfast, although day by day he became more depressed.

> "I told him that Jesus loved me and didn't heal me, and that Jesus loved him and might not heal him either. Two weeks later the nurse called and said Joe was ready to discuss his disability and how to live with it. I went back to see Joe and help him learn the tricks of the trade, how to be self sufficient from a wheelchair."

REALITY

Full reality is usually slow in arriving, and perhaps that is a good thing. How many of us could have accepted the full load of reality of all the consequences and limitations of our diagnosis in one lump? Reality must be handled like the huge rock pile on most farms—one rock at a time. If you were asked to remove one of those huge piles you most likely would say it could not be done. But it was put there by only one or two individuals—one rock at a time. And that is the way most of us must face reality—one rock at a time.

Again, because we are all individuals, there is no precise prescription for handling the load forced upon us by reality. What works for one may not work for another. However, there is a universal premise that when faithfully practiced does work. It is that of having a positive áttitude toward any of the consequences and limitations of our diagnosis.

Norman Vincent Peale's book, *The Power of Positive Thinking*, as well as Dr. Robert Schuller's emphasis on positive thinking on his TV program, "Hour of Power," are not out of step with today's research.

> "Disease-fighting cells can both produce and respond to the same chemicals that brain cells use to communicate with one another. Studies have shown that immune-system cells can be weakened by mental attitudes." (Journal of Personality and Social Psychology)

This does not mean having a "Pollyanna" approach where one says, "Oh, isn't it wonderful that I have this malady." It does mean that we look at some of the positive aspects and say to ourselves, "It could have been much worse; in fact, many good things have come out of the bad."

In my case there were a number of good things coming from my limitations that have given some satisfactions that most likely would have eluded me had I been left in one good piece. When the negative begins to draw power from my life I search out the positive. One of those positive aspects of my paralysis by polio is that it slowed me down to a point where I could smell the flowers. In my first 18 years I had only two speeds—wide open and sleeping. My mobility, slowed down to a creep, has given me the opportunity to see and savor many things that would have otherwise escaped me.

That means the minute observation of nature while sitting at one of our camp sights when most everyone in our group has trudged off into the woods. It means people-watching in the mall (great sport for a psychologist). It means time to think creatively and explore complex and controversial ideas. It means there is time to listen to myself and to you. And most of all it has given me a life-long profession for both study and experience in the world of disability. It means that my limitations gave me the opportunity to talk to you as is happening at this moment. Truly, this privilege is cherished and gives me a feeling of contribution to humanity. Without polio it could not have happened.

DEPRESSION

What more could possibly be said about depression than what is readily available on the market? Once again the important aspect of depression is to recognize it for what it is—a possible chemically-induced malfunction of the emotions from drugs or genes, and/or a normal reaction of the emotions to the fact and feeling of a loss. Did we suffer a loss when we became the apparent victim of our disease or condition? You bet your sweet bottom we did. In the passing of a few seconds some of us lost our mobility, our jobs, our spouse and/or families, our self esteem, and our life-time goals. Some of us lost everything but our very existence on the face of this earth. Shouldn't we be depressed?

Unfortunately, depression thrives upon itself. It appears that we are going to discover more and more that depression has a chemical basis—that our thought processes trigger a chemical reaction. Remember the article quoted on page 7 in the segment on Reality? If the brain responds chemically to depression or negative thoughts, how can we break the cycle or snow-ball effect of getting deeper and deeper into depression?

It is not as easy as some would suggest, that you just tell the person to get off or out of it. An angry face-off is not the prescription for curing depression. If there were any absolute cut-dried-and-tried methods, its discoverers would be rich. There would be no need for therapy nor for anyone to have a "down" day. It would be heaven on earth. At this moment there is no cure.

However, there are some ways to combat it. Depression cannot live without food. Negative thoughts are food on which depression thrives. About the only advice I can give persons suffering from depression is to quit feeding it. Thinking and brooding—wallowing in our troubles—is the arch-enemy of mental health. Unfortunately, the person with a disability often has too much thinking time. The disability prevents utilizing normal healing methods such as hitting a golf ball around a course or other physical activities to divert one's attention from the problems.

If some types of depression are within the control of our minds, who controls our minds? Can't we choose to think of pleasant memories or happy things? We cannot be induced into a hypnotic trance unless we allow it. Someone can possess our bodies (such as prisoners of war), but our minds can only be possessed with our permission. Therefore, we have the power and ability to choose to think positive or negative thoughts—the power to feed or starve our depression. "Oh, sure," you say. "You make it sound so easy. Have you ever tried to practice what you preach?"

Well, yes. And you are right, it was not as easy as it sounds. My personality, as luck would have it, is by nature quite up and optimistic. That doesn't make me better or worse than you, but it does give an edge in being successful in dealing with depression. Let me tell you my most disturbing depression.

It was shortly after we had moved to Phoenix in 1973. Our move had been prompted by what was diagnosed as traumatic arthritis from overuse of arms in lifting my body and wheeling my chair. Although the diagnosis turned out rather to be post-polio syndrome, it was nonetheless extremely limiting. It prevented much wheeling and offered a number of falls when pain encompassed my joints during a transfer to toilet, bed, car, or whatever.

For the first time in my post-polio life, I was forced to stop all major physical activity. Many hours were spent in my recliner just thinking about life—my life. What was going to happen to me? How about my family? That's right, my poor family, I thought. I began thinking about Janice, my wife, who married me "like this" and had never had one day of what one could consider a normal marriage. Sure, married to a wheelchair. And how about our children? They had never known a father who could play ball or other sports with them. My wife and children all had been cheated by my disability, and now it was worse, and who knew how much worse it would become?

As I reviewed my past, present, and future life, sitting in that recliner, something happened to my otherwise up-and-optimistic outlook. For the first time in my life I became depressed, and the more depressed I became, the deeper I sank into depression. The depression was obvious to me, and from a professional position it should have been easily handled. After all, didn't I have all the answers for others?

The bottom of the depressive cycle came when after brooding several months, the logical conclusion was that my family—those I loved the most and for whom I would give my life—would be better off without this drag of a husband and father. Am I speaking of suicide? Yes, I am. The person who had discussed suicide with many of his clients was now experiencing for the first time what others with those thoughts face.

As you may have guessed, it didn't happen. I did take myself and my mind into hand and took my own advice. When those negative thoughts would try to permeate my defenses I would turn to positive thoughts. My wife had a husband who loved her more than anything in this world. He had provided her with love, companionship, and stability in a marriage relationship. She was my best friend as well as my wife. She had never grumbled about being married to a "cripple." There was no evidence in any way that our children were scarred or suffered from my disability. As I looked for positive thoughts they kept tumbling out.

It took many months to rid myself of those frightening (and I do mean frightening) thoughts about suicide. When I finally had the courage I told Janice and we discussed how I felt about her and the children. She looked at me and shook her head in unbelief, "Did you ever ask me how I felt about being *stuck* with you? You owed me that, the kids that, and you owed it to yourself. Have you any idea what your faulty thinking would have done to us if you had carried out your ideas?" No, but later I recognized that suicide can be the most selfish act a person can commit.

BITTERNESS/ANGER

One time an auto-parts counterman blurted out to me, "Are you very bitter?" Another time in a class seminar on disability I was asked by a student, "Are you bitter?" Those of us with disabilities are automatically ascribed bitterness, or at least the "ordinary" world expects us to be bitter. Often when receiving a referral from another agency, the social worker will say, "It is so unfortunate that this person is so bitter."

It seems to be expected of us, so what is wrong with being bitter? Now it is not a grave sin to be bitter for it is no more unusual than denial, fantasy, reality, and depression. Bitterness is not the problem; it is that some of us get hung up on it too long—some for life. The problem with bitterness is that it colors all aspects of thoughts and behavior. If it is allowed to continue it will distort our view of our world and of ourselves. Long-term bitterness is non-productive.

Not long ago at a seminar for the disabled, anger became a topic of conversation. In the professional world there is an all-out offensive against anger. One day there was a referral from a social worker at a local hospital. He had a patient who was disabled and who had tried to commit suicide (oops, we are back on that subject). "She is so full of anger over her disability, and it is our hope that you can help her dissipate the anger."

By the time my schedule allowed a visit, she had been discharged from the hospital so a home visit was in order. What a delightful person she was. Her disability had cost her a great deal: first, it was the loss of her studies and desire to be a medical doctor; then it was the ability to do anything for herself; and finally it almost cost her life.

She, her family, and I talked freely over the attempted suicide and how she felt about life. She was angry and it showed. Finally, I told her that the hospital social worker had recommended that we work on dissipating her anger. We both laughed. That was the last thing I wanted her to lose. Rather, that anger needed to be redirected toward living rather than dying. That anger (not bitterness) had the potential to give her fuel to propel herself through each day. Without it she would have given up.

While bitterness is always negative, anger can be positive. If Lee Iacocca had gone to a counselor and had been told that his anger at Henry Ford II for firing him must be addressed because it was destructive, it is doubtful there would be a Chrysler Corporation today. It was the anger Mr. Iacocca had for the treatment received from Ford that motivated him to facilitate one of the biggest corporate turnarounds in industrial history. Had he seen a counselor who did not understand the value of anger, perhaps I would never have had the pleasure of owning and driving a Plymouth minivan, a great vehicle for a wheelchair user.

So there we see the positive side of anger. Let yourself be angry. If you find yourself coming to the boiling point, blow off a little steam in a manner in which others (so often those you love) are not burned. Regardless of what the current philosophy is on anger, it can be controlled and it should be. Anger out of control and/or misdirected is dangerous.

How thankful I am for a mother who taught me that being angry was okay, but being angry out of control was not. In her terminology, when I "flew off the handle," there was discipline administered. Believe me, I do have a temper but no one has ever seen it in full fury. Learning how to control it has made my professional and personal life much more productive. When the office personnel would hear a client call me every dirty name in the book and sometimes even threaten my life, they would shake their heads and ask, "How do you manage to keep calm?" Thanks, Mom, for the lessons in control.

Fear

Somewhere during these emotional steps, usually as our naiveté fades and we begin to face reality, we become frightened over the prospects of our diagnosis. We fear the consequences of the physical and/or mental limits that have been dumped on us—some that are obvious and some that we just anticipate.

We fear what will happen to all our dreams and goals of work, play, and companionship. The insurance TV commercials pry at our fear such as the one where the older man hobbles along and is forced to sit down. He rubs his legs and then looks up at his wife and says, "I don't want to be a burden to you." None of us want to be a burden to anyone, including ourselves—and it is a legitimate fear.

Rather than discussing the individual fears that each of you might face, let us take a more general approach. Let's look at the phenomenon of fear itself. Remember the oft-quoted words of Franklin Roosevelt in his 1933 inaugural address? "The only fear we have is fear itself." That is what I would like to impress upon you at this moment—we should fear FEAR. Fear, in itself, has never solved anything, and it can paralyze our thinking.

So often we see those newly diagnosed with multiple sclerosis reading and uncovering the variety of symptoms of the disorder: double vision, loss of balance, tremors, numbness, and many more. Fearfully and anxiously they retreat to a corner of life and wait for each of those insidious symptoms to appear. What a tragedy!

The medical books don't tell them that although this is the medical list of all the symptoms, that *all* people do not have *all* the symptoms. Some may have only one, perhaps two. They may have a remission of that symptom for months or years. No one can predict which symptoms a person with MS will have nor their severity or duration.

What a waste of time it is to cower in a corner waiting for disaster that may never come. The old adage, "Don't cross the bridge until you come to it," is excellent advice. So often I see persons with a progressively-worsening disease or condition just sit back and fearfully wait out the supposed impending disaster.

My fear for so many of you is that you will allow your "diagnosis" to possess you. Just because you have multiple sclerosis, cerebral palsy, muscular dystrophy, cystic fibrosis, or whatever, does not mean that multiple sclerosis, polio, or whatever, needs to have you. I had polio; it does not have me. You may have MS, MD, CA, CF, SCI, ALS, and all the other letters of the alphabet, but they do not necessarily have you unless you permit it. Don't let your disease or condition be the biggest thing in your life. Don't let it occupy every thought and conversation you have. Don't go to sleep thinking about it and don't wake up thinking about it. Be its master and not its slave. This is not easy or simple, but it can be done.

So often these words are unheeded, but it is my hope that my life could underscore that statement. Granted, my limitations may not be the same or as severe as many of yours, but you must face the challenge of your limitations with whatever skills you possess as I must face with my skills. What you should know is that a severe disability does not necessarily have to remove you from life. It may change your course a bit, but you don't need to quit paddling.

CHALLENGES

However, if your circumstances so dictate and you find yourself attempting to paddle your canoe in the mainstream of life, know that it will wring out of you every ounce of the stuff from which you are made. It will push you to the wall of exhaustion and you may be tempted to give up and drift backwards with the current. Know that competing in a whole world with only a part of a body is demanding and dangerous.

Those of us who have the worn-out bodies of twenty or thirty years of competition in a *whole* world know what we are talking about. Pushing yourself to the brink of physical and/or mental disaster might look good to your neighbors, family, and friends, but the long-term results can be disastrous.

How many "gimpy" athletes are limping around in life nursing an "old football" or other such injury? "A few moments or a few years of glory should not be exchanged for a lifetime of limitation and pain," you say. And you are right, but let's apply the same principle to ourselves. We must learn to pace ourselves. We must not be goaded by the world of spectators of disability into pushing harder and harder, higher and higher.

Some of those in the professional world of rehabilitation have castigated me for even suggesting that we think about slacking off. "You give them an excuse to be lazy," they say. My reply is that those who are looking for an excuse will find one. If not mine, there will be another, perhaps of their own making. It is my contention that those who really need an excuse to slow down should have the opportunity of evaluating the long-term destructive forces of being driven to the extreme either by their own drive or the encouragement of others.

Somewhere along the line a popular philosophy has developed that you can be anything you want to be, and you can do anything you want to do. All you have to do is want it badly enough and struggle hard enough and it will be yours. Someone once snorted at me, "If you really wanted to walk you could have if you had tried hard enough." Oh, horse hockey! Had I not known better at the time, that silly statement could have been very emotionally destructive to me.

Too often I see the friends and families of persons who are disabled try to motivate the person beyond all good sense. "Well, reach for the stars, and if you don't make it and have to take less, nothing is lost." What a crock! All the disabled person most likely will learn from this failure is that he has disappointed those who had faith in him and who encouraged him.

Encouragement we need, but not toward impossible goals such as reaching for the stars. The problem is that most persons do not comprehend which are reasonable and which are unreasonable goals. You would not believe some of the outlandish goals professionals have held out to the disabled. Some they knew were impossible but were nonetheless used as motivational bait. Others were thought probable, but were presented as possible. To these goals, anything less than success was considered a cop out.

My clients would often come into my office and tell me of some goal that may or may not have been possible. Who was I to say what a person could or could not accomplish? Too often in my early rehabilitation days I had been told that some task or goal was impossible for me, but I accomplished it anyway. It became my philosophy that every person has a right to fail on his own. It was not my prerogative to tell any person that he would never be able to do the pole vault sitting in a wheelchair. That discovery must come from within that person.

The sensible approach was not to think high, but to think low. Rather than a designed failure that would be destructive, make a list of steps needed for success and then take each small step until failure. In this way failure was not destructive because the person had built up a series of successes to that point of failure.

When someone came to me after a devastating experience with failure, we began something like this: "Now just suppose that I could walk and that I wanted to jump this hurdle. You walked over and put it on the highest pins and told me to run and jump. Each trial brought failure. What would you tell me to do?" In almost every case they answered, "Lower the hurdle." What tremendous insight we have when we are not emotionally involved.

Rather than lower the hurdle a pin or two, we discussed the procedure and decided to lower it to the point of obvious success and then repeat the jumps and raise the bar until we could no longer clear it. Then we would lower the bar and work on perfecting our jump with an occasional try at the higher level.

Why can't we learn to do this with all goals? We have been erroneously goaded into believing that we must set our sights higher than our abilities (reach for the stars) so that we will not sell ourselves short of reaching our highest point. Keep in mind that success motivates, failure devastates.

Sources Of Help

There are three sources of help: 1) self, spouse, and other family members, 2) community resources such as health agencies with their vast array of services that include support groups, and 3) your own personal religious/spiritual beliefs.

The greatest source of help that is immediately within your grasp is naturally your own self. In making demands of yourself in these times of deep need, keep in mind that the self does have real limits, not just imaginary ones as some might suggest. There is a limit to what we can demand of ourselves. There are countless books on the market that promote self motivation. They have been written by M.D.s, Ph.D.s and others with lesser credentials. It should be understood that many of these books and philosophies are borderline to full-blown extremism and that very few persons, if any, are really able to make them work. You say, "Well, they can't hurt you, can they?" Yes, in a sense that you may see yourself as a failure when you don't achieve the advertised results. Losing faith in one's self promotes depression.

In many cases the next most important source of help and strength is your spouse. However, we must keep in mind that in the case of disability, the spouse is also going through a deep crisis and has needs as well. You must learn to lean upon each other's strengths as well as to accept each other's weaknesses. There are times when one of you will be up and the other down, then vice versa. And unfortunately, there are times when you will both be down together. However, even in weakness we can lean on each other. Then we must acknowledge that there are times when a spouse cannot help, and sometimes a spouse can actually be a detriment because there is a lack of understanding, commitment, or love in a relationship. In that case they become a part of the problem and not the part of the solution. All persons are not capable of handling a disability, their own or another's.

Then there are other family members such as parents. If you have your own children, would you not give up your life for them if it became necessary? Most of you would, so why would your parents at any age not be expected to be vitally interested in your diagnosis and progress in either your improving or becoming worse? Stubbornness keeps many of us from allowing those who kissed the bleeding knee in our childhood from kissing our cheek in our adult hurts. Do not keep those who love you in darkness. Tell them how you feel and how you are doing. Parents have a sixth sense when it comes to interpreting how their children are doing and feeling. Saying you are doing fine when you are not does not put them at ease, it confuses them. Unfortunately, distance often limits the help we can receive from parents and other family members who live apart from us.

You will notice that children were not included in the sources of help. Why? If your children are under the age of twenty-five, they are most likely too busy with the selfish interests of childhood. Perhaps one of the deepest hurts I hear is this: "My children don't appear to be concerned about me. Sometimes they seem to do everything to disturb me. Don't they care about me? Can't they see I need their help?" No, they generally do not see others' needs, even the deep needs of their parents. It is not because they are bad, insensitive, or unloving; it is because they are children. Yes, they care about you in their own childish/selfish way. Often they become angry with you because you no longer can serve them as you did in the past. If they are over twenty-five, they are most likely too busy with their own lives and families. Although they cannot comprehend the ramifications of your diagnosis, they hate what has happened but they do not know how to express their anger or on whom it should be directed. No, few persons will find their children as a source of help. Even though this might be the rule, we must acknowledge that there are exceptions.

One of the great sources of help may come from the health agency that specializes in your particular disability or disease. No one person or agency can know it all. There is too much to know about every disease or condition, so it makes good sense to single out a condition or disease (or related groups) and concentrate on knowing as much as possible about that problem. These health agencies are usually listed in the Yellow Pages of your phone directory under the heading, Social Service Organizations. Most will be found alphabetically listed according to the diagnosis. There are some exceptions for those who work with more than one type of disability, such as Easter Seals. If an agency cannot help you, most all of these social service organizations are equipped to refer you to the organization best suited to your needs.

The health agency that specializes in your problem will keep up with research and treatment methods. It will direct you to counselors, support groups, or other community resources. One of the great discoveries in associating yourself with your special health agency is that you are not alone. You have the company of thousands of others in like circumstances. It is to your advantage to associate yourself with them and benefit from the experiences of others. You also have the opportunity of contributing what you have experienced with those less experienced. It is a time of learning and sharing. Keep in mind that your health agency needs you just as much as you need it.

Finally, God gets last place as a source of help because this is common practice with us humans, just as it is to read the instructions after everything else has failed. All too often God gets put up on the shelf and hears from us only when disaster strikes, and then only after we have come to the end of our rope.

Back in 1972 a rehabilitation expert made this statement at a seminar I was attending: "I believe the deepest need of the handicapped person today is a spiritual need." That remark captured my attention, first because I believed he was correct, and second because he had the fortitude to express it. So often we convince ourselves that any thought or statement relating to religion is so private that it cannot or should not be mentioned, and certainly not by a professional person who is not a member of the clergy. And even clergymen are cautioned to keep silence in a captive, non-voluntary audience.

It is not my intention at this point to attempt to convince anyone that there is a God or to discuss or try to express or convert you to any of my spiritual beliefs. However, if you have become disillusioned with your religion or too busy to be spiritually minded, it is my intent to ask you to search for the God of your youth. Go back into time and pick up your religion where you left it. Try to discover or rediscover the tenets of your faith that will give you the help you need. For those of you who are unchurched, please believe me when I tell you that the understanding of God and eternity (within our human limits) can be a mighty force in restructuring our thinking. When all else fails, try God. Or better yet, don't wait; get God involved now.

A New Sense Of Direction

Many have said to me that they knew that they could not handle a disability (or a long-term illness). My reply is that no person can predict his reaction to a "diagnosis" until that situation is actually faced. In many situations of adjusting to a disability or diagnosis, those thought to be strong often fall and those thought to be weak often prevail.

When our daughter, Leanne, was about fourteen years of age, she and I happened to watch a movie on television together. It was titled, "*Leave Yesterday Behind*," and it was about a man (played by John Ritter) who had become paralyzed in a horse accident. At the end of the movie we sat for a moment in silence until she broke it by asking, "Daddy, will you make me a promise?" Good sense dictates that one does not promise what one does not know, so I told her to spell it out first and then I would answer.

I was somewhat startled by her request: "Daddy, would you promise me that if anything like that ever happened to me that you would somehow find a way to kill me? I know that I could not handle anything like that." My response was this: "No, you can't know if you could or could not handle it until it happened. And besides, where would you be if your father had felt like that?" Today, twenty years later my professional guess is that she is capable of coping with most anything that comes along in life. I just hope nothing comes along in her life to test this.

Another statement often heard is this: "I am not handling this *diagnosis* very well." My reply is, "And how do you know that you are not? Do you have any standard by which you can judge how well you are doing?" Of course there are no standards published to evaluate your emotional rehabilitation progress other than those emotional steps to recovery mentioned earlier. You cannot evaluate your own "handling" unless you have had vast experience in observing the performance of others in similar circumstances.

If you are looking for a timetable of adjustment, it is my experience with myself and others that the average person needs from three to eight years to adjust to a traumatic disease or condition. In the case of unstable or changing limitations, the adjustment period can last as long as life itself. Don't for one minute think you can say to yourself and others, "I can conquer this. Just give me a week or so of getting myself together and a little time to cry and I'll be okay." Of course you can conquer it, but know that it will not be overnight.

It is my hope (yes, and my prayer) that this chapter will contribute to the understanding and restructuring of any of the areas of your life that have been changed or challenged by a "diagnosis." Now that you have information that can help dispel the darkness surrounding your "diagnosis," it is time for you to get on with your life. If it means getting on with life in a wheelchair or whatever, do it!

LIFE IS YOUR MOST PRECIOUS COMMODITY—DO NOT WASTE IT.

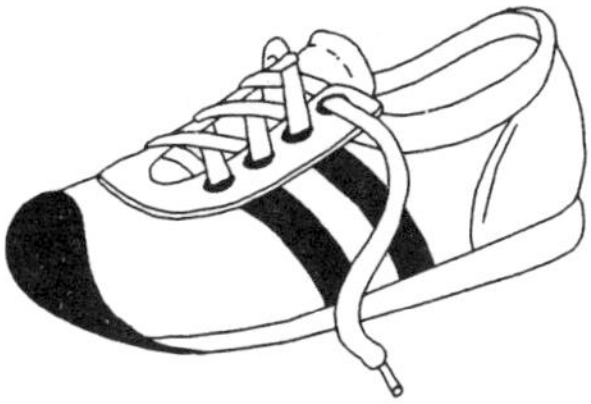

Chapter 2

PARENTS OF HANDICAPPED CHILDREN

THE THUNDERSTORMS OF LIFE

If your "child" is newborn or fifty years of age, this chapter should have meaning for you. In his book, *The Road Less Traveled*, M. Scott Peck, M.D., wrote:

> "Life is difficult. This is one of the greatest truths.... Most do not fully see this truth that life is difficult. Instead they moan more or less incessantly, noisily or subtly, about the enormity of their problems, their burdens, and their difficulties as if life were generally easy, as if life should be easy."

Bumper-sticker reading is a driving pastime of mine as they tell a good deal about the driver or owner of the automobile. However, sometimes it takes some tricky driving to get close enough to read one that looks interesting. One such sticker affixed on the bumper of a beat-up car caught my attention because of the general rudeness of the driver. My reward came at the next traffic light which turned red for the driver and I could conveniently pull up behind her. There, blazoned in black one-inch letters was this message:

LIFE IS A BITCH, AND SO AM I

The message that "life is a bitch" bounced around my mind for a few weeks. Perhaps from my unusual perch of working intensely with disability and with disabled persons for forty-some years gave credibility to the message. Oh, sure, I know that "into each life some rain must fall," but why do some persons and families reap a tornado and others only a nice drizzle during a dry spell? However, we all know that in the end no one escapes all the miseries of life, for ultimately a person whom we love very much will be hurt by life or by death. When we finally have had enough experience in living even the best life possible, we are forced to conclude that life at its best is not all that great.

In the *Bible* the book of Job aptly decries the state of man in relation to life's difficulties. You perhaps remember the story of the righteous man, Job, who was beset with every misery possible, from the loss of all material wealth to the death of his children, including pain and suffering in his own body. What a truism when Job philosophized: "*Yet man is born unto trouble, as the sparks fly upward.*" (Job 5:7) It is comforting that the story began with a character reference for Job, that he was perfect and upright, and one who feared God and hated evil. Without this bit of understanding many would conclude that Job was a bad man who got in life what he had coming to him.

Therefore, not only is life difficult, it is also unfair. When attempting to understand unforeseen, unavoidable, unhappy, or devastating happenings in our lives or that of another, we have all heard the statement, "Life is not fair." Many times I have agreed with a statement from a friend or counselee who stammered, "It isn't fair!" Nowhere is there a promise that it would be for you, for me, or for anyone else. No, life is not fair nor has it ever been fair.

So often these devastating happenings come out of the sky and strike us like a bolt of lightning. Few persons really understand the potential for disaster that is in a single, even small bolt of lightning. Lightning kills and disables thousands of Americans each year, yet we move from day to day feeling no impending threat of being struck down suddenly by a thunderous bolt of lightning. Being struck by lightning is not as uncommon as most persons think. Neither is it as uncommon for a child to be born with physical or mental complications, for as many as one child in every hundred births has some type of disability or birth defect.

Although you know it is common, how prepared are you for the devastation of a true strike of lightning in your life today or tomorrow? Can one prepare himself for such a thing? No. Why, then, do we castigate ourselves for being ill prepared for the event of disability in the life of our child?

Who is responsible? When lightning damages a tree or person, or ignites a raging forest fire, do we not use the term "act of God" to assess blame? When someone is born into this world with a handicap (or acquires one later in life), do we not by nature attempt to assess blame? *"Master, who did sin, this man or his parents, that he was born blind?"* (John 9:2). Christ answered in the following verse *"Neither hath this man sinned, nor his parents...."* Those disciples made the same error that continues to this day, that of trying to assess blame in the case of disability. Don't be caught in this human trap of blaming yourself or God.

It seems so logical: for every effect there must be a cause. If God isn't to blame, and certainly no right-thinking person could blame the child, there is only one other logical culprit—we, the parents must in some way, great or small, be responsible. It seems unthinkable that in today's world of answers there cannot be an answer to the "whys" of disability. And my answer to your unanswerable question is that deep feelings of personal guilt are normal—and most often are unfounded and must be discarded.

When we read of a person or group of persons being struck by lightning, we shake our heads and go on to the next news item. It is much the same when we hear or read of someone being disabled from an accidental happening, birth defect, disease, the aging process, natural response to genetic heritage, or a faulty body from misuse.

What we can learn from the strike of a lightning bolt is (1) that it is completely controlled by the laws of electron movement—the laws of nature; (2) that it is not a respecter of persons (it is not fair); (3) that it often comes with no warning and it often results in immediate death or disability; (4) and that society as a whole is not concerned with the devastation it may cause in your life.

Please don't read into this that no one cares. There are many caring individuals (trusting that I am one of these) who care, but society as a mass is unconcerned unless the lightning strikes them or those they love. Perhaps this lack of concern is an emotional survival mechanism in the human being, for if we were to be intensely concerned with all the strikes of lightning in all the lives of all the people on earth, would we not go berserk? Therefore, let us realize that for the most part, with the exception of a few caring people, we will be forced to bear our devastation primarily alone.

Primarily alone—however, not totally alone, for without support nothing and no one can stand. Support is a scientific law of physics, and support is also a psychological law. To survive a crisis we must have some base of support—family, friends, and others. This is why support groups are so vital in coping with disability. Along with the needed support, the group offers information and advice from the heart rather than from the textbooks.

When we are ready to accept that life in general is difficult, that life is not fair, and that in our difficulty and unfair circumstance we are not guilty nor are we totally alone, then we are ready to face our individual devastation with determination and reality. It is my hope that these pages will offer you some direction, comfort, and challenge to face the lightning strike in your life, that of a disability of someone you love dearly.

Beating The Odds

That bolt of lightning from out of nowhere in my life presented itself when I was eighteen years of age, that time in life when young persons believe their bodies to be indestructible. There was no warning other than a severe headache for several days along with a backache that finally engulfed my entire body, then paralysis and a 13-month hospital stay. It was then and continues to be the greatest challenge of my life, that is to live as normal a life as possible under my individual circumstances and limitations. My life has been one of frustrating competition with able-bodied persons—a four-cylinder engine competing in an eight-cylinder world.

In many cases success stories of disabled persons hinder more than help those who are struggling on the bottom rungs of the ladder. For every story of success there are hundreds or even thousands who cannot claim any great human success. We don't hear much about those who fail and it gives a false impression that all one has to do is want to succeed, give it their best shot, and it will happen. If failure is the result, it is because the person didn't want success badly enough or they didn't put enough effort into it.

Success for anyone is a very individual matter. It is more than just struggling to reach the top of the ladder or even the next rung. It is made up of who and what we are in relation to our circumstances. Most often our success is a team effort rather than the single-player effort. In whatever success I have enjoyed it must be realized that only a part of my success was because of any drive or direction that was my personal possession.

First of all, I came from a kind and loving family from whom I received every ounce of support within their resources. My wife is also a kind, loving, and devoted person. Since our marriage in 1949 most of my success can be credited to her. My drive and direction would have come to naught were it not for early family support and later from my wife. How then can persons say to another that if you do what they did or if you follow their example or pattern you will succeed? (That also includes seminars on "How to Become a Millionaire.") Your children cannot do what I did nor can anyone else, simply because they are not me or "anyone else."

Through no fault or genius of our own, we struggle through life with what we have. When we were born we came equipped with whatever intellectual and emotional accessories we were to have in this life. This does not mean that what we have cannot be enhanced. Your child's life and accomplishments can be a rewarding experience. Although self-feeding, shoe tying, potty training, along with all the other developmental tasks, might be months or years behind "other" children, does that make that success any less rewarding? No—more so!

One of my friends with cerebral palsy told of learning to ride a tricycle—at the age of twelve.

> "My mother could not watch. I was determined even though I could not pedal nor keep my balance. I fell off time after time. Scabs and screams were a part of my learning, but one day it happened. It took five years, but I did it! I did it!"

Not only did she master the tricycle, she mastered the demands of the University of Minnesota, the demands of a wife, and finally the demands of motherhood.

Darlene was a delightful young woman in her mid-thirties. Cerebral palsy restricted her mobility to a wheelchair. Although her speech was slow, it was very understandable. In my effort to determine if speech improvement in CP took place after the teens, I asked her if her speech had improved after high school. "Bob, if you had heard me speak when I was eighteen, you would not have been able to understand me." At that moment it came to me that at no time in life can we give up—on our children or on ourselves. Success has no time limits.

After many years in the counseling profession, it has finally dawned upon me that to be a successful counselor I must help the person work with what he has, not what I have. Therefore, in this sense there can be no such thing as failure because there is no set standard for success. Only the persons who are trying can make the judgment that they did or are doing all within their power.

Should I feel like a failure because there is no desire in me to wheel my wheelchair from coast to coast, or for even 10 or 100 miles? Should you feel you have failed if your disabled child's progress does not meet the expectations of the school system, your physician's, or your own goals? Falling short of a goal should not be assessed as failure; however, failing to give it "your best shot" *is* failure. No one other than the individual himself can assess failure. You cannot say I have failed, and I cannot say you have failed. So let's put this success/failed assessment into proper perspective.

Fight Or Surrender

Several years ago there was an article in the newspaper regarding eccentrics accompanied by a checklist. It was so interesting that I stuck it on our cork board. Several days later while musing the subject, my question to Janice, my wife, was whether she viewed me as an eccentric. She first gazed at the ceiling, then marched over and took the article off the cork board and then walked over and faced me with it.

She began the checklist and after each statement that included such statements as "A loner, Doesn't care what others think," etc., she looked at me for a moment and then drawled, "Yyyyessss." The last check-list statement was, "Hard to get along with." At least there was one factor that didn't line me up with eccentrics.

I waited for her to say, "No, Dear, at least you are not difficult to get along with." But to my surprise and hurt she drawled another "Yyyyessss." After a few seconds of thought she said, "No, I take that back (long pause—and I felt relief until she continued); I think of you more as a challenge." Now she could have surrendered to whatever it is that makes me difficult to live with, but she chose to fight—to see my rough spots as a challenge.

Our personality dictates how each of us looks at life as a whole as well as individual situations in life. On the ends of the scale there are the extreme optimists and the extreme pessimists. Most of us fall somewhere in between. That reminds me of the story of the brothers (perhaps like the *Bible* story of Joseph and his brothers). The older brothers were jealous of the attention their younger brother received from their parents. It was Christmas and all the boys hung up their stockings by the fireplace. One brother had a wonderful idea for a dirty trick: they would go out to the barn and get horse manure and fill the youngest's sock.

When Christmas morning came the boys dashed downstairs, the older ones held back to watch the fun. The little guy grabbed his sock and peered into it looking for the goodies only to see (and smell) the manure. Rather than the reward of disappointment the trick-players had hoped for, the youngest beamed with excitement. "Hey, you guys," he exploded, "I had a pony but he got away." And so it is with life, some of us can see a pony in a pile of manure.

Still fresh in my mind is the phone call from a distraught mother whose thirty-year-old daughter was degenerating rapidly from multiple sclerosis. For the first time in my memory someone could not be convinced that a counseling session with me might help. "No, you can't help me—you cannot change things." There was no question that no one could change her daughter's condition or prognosis, but my plea was to at least give it a chance for a new approach. She had nothing to lose, even money, for the counseling would be free of charge. Although I could not change her circumstances, perhaps together we could develop a new look or attitude toward her problems. "No, you can't help me nor can anyone else," she ended our conversation and hung up. My heart ached for her, but there was nothing that could be done. How I wished that a little pony could be injected into that horse manure in her life.

Recently I met a mother who within less than a year had both of her teenage children become quadriplegics, one also being severely brain damaged. Her son became a quadriplegic in an accident. Six months later she received a call to come immediately to the hospital. She was prepared for some emergency with him, but discovered when she arrived at the hospital emergency room that it was her daughter who had been involved in an accident.

It is easy to become distraught over your own disability or your one child who is physically and/or mentally impaired. Could you cope with two or four in a similar condition? Most likely, whatever we can come up with in the way of personal devastation, it could be topped. If comparing our situation with one worse would automatically change our outlook, then all we would have to do is compile a long list of severe personal tragedies and have it presented to us.

This is often illustrated in the statement about the man who felt sorry for himself for having no shoes until *he saw* the man who had no feet. It is a mistake for either a professional counselor, family member, or a friend to attempt to drive home a new insight or attitude by comparing the plight with someone who has it so much worse. There are numerous situations that could be written from my mind and files that are far worse than what you and I are facing. Shoving them in our faces will not change our outlook. No, we cannot drive a new outlook into another person.

Most of the disability in our lives cannot be changed, or at least changed very much. However it is possible to change our look at the situation. How can that be done successfully? It is truly the power of positive thinking. Without going into personal detail, believe me when I tell you that focusing on the "can dos" rather than the "can't dos" makes the difference. Negatives cannot be denied, but they can certainly be tucked into a corner.

If we can't drive or force a new and positive attitude into another person, what can we do? Well, for one thing we can lay eggs. The hen only lays the egg; its hatching is dependent on fertilization and continual warmth and turning. Attitudes, concepts or ideas, like eggs can be laid. Chicken hens do not lay chickens; they lay eggs. And like eggs, attitudes and concepts require warmth, movement, and time to incubate. When an attitude adjustment is in order in either a parent or the disabled child, try laying an egg—a soft suggestion in that person's nest (mind).

There are times in my counsel when words are of no value. We can play with the psyche for hours with no results, as in one case in which I did just that. It was months later upon a chance meeting with that person that he said, "It was not until you left me and I secretly watched you struggle to get yourself and your wheelchair into the car that I realized how fortunate I was. Since that time I have a new look and understanding of my disability."

As age creeps over me and the "post polio syndrome" continues its dirty work on me, there are times when anger wells up in my soul over these new limitations (loss of strength, muscle and joint pain, fatigue, and the other "delights" of the syndrome). For the first time in my life I had to take myself in hand and say, "Hey, I know many quads who would give most anything to have one of your hands or even 10% of your hand function. There are countless others who would be delighted to be able to sit 16 hours a day in a wheelchair even with the pain."

It worked! Why? Because it came from within me and not from someone else. Don't try to minimize my disability by maximizing others. You must let me do that all by myself. There is no magic or set rules. The new look at disability comes often as sudden insight, early or perhaps late in life. For that reason we can never give up that this change can take place.

It's Okay To Cry

"It is okay to cry," I said to myself as the tears rolled down my face. It was shortly after being released from isolation (polio is a contagious virus for two weeks after onset). In naiveté and wonderment, lying in a ward with nine other men who were similarly afflicted by polio, I cried quietly to myself and to God. Nights were long and radios filled the silence of our souls into the wee hours of the mornings.

It was one of those late nights that with immense effort I managed to tug the covers over my head for privacy. For the first and last time came tears related to my losses from polio. The callouses from normal walking and working were yet on my feet. This was a new and fearful experience trying to move and having nothing happen. Not only was walking impossible, so was sitting up or even rolling over in bed. My tears spilled from a heart that simply said, "Why, God, why this?" Each of the men in that ward grieved over a loss—the loss of a whole and functioning body. One man was also grieving the loss of his wife who left him because of his disability. Each had his individual griefs. Yes, it was okay to cry—for any one of us.

There has been more written and studies done on grieving than perhaps any other subject. It is there for those who have lost a husband, a wife, a child, a parent, or even a pet. But seldom do we see anything written on grieving over the loss of one's body parts or functions even though our elderly population is in constant grief over these month-by-month and year-by-year losses.

Neither do we find much written on grieving over the loss of something that never was ours to lose—that is, we never had our hands on it. What a loss it is to a parent who excitedly expects and awaits the birth of a normal child only to have the doctor or hospital social worker say to them in a quiet and sympathetic tone, "I am sorry to have to tell you this, but your child has a *few* problems." It can be a tremendous loss—the loss of a dream.

My mother heard those frightening words from the doctor, "I'm sorry, but I am afraid the boy has polio." Later my parents were informed that I would never walk again, and perhaps not even be able to sit up. They came almost daily to the hospital to visit me in those early months. Later they told me that those visits usually ended in tears in the hallway or while driving home—tears that I never saw. Did they lose something? You answer that for yourself, especially if you are a parent. They lost their dreams for me that most parents have for their children. They also shared with me the physical pain of the disease. It devastated our family, but we all recovered in time.

My family lost something as did I. We certainly can lose things that were never truly ours to hold. My losses of dreams from paralysis cannot compare with the loss of a dream for a normal child, but nonetheless it gives me a right and an understanding to talk from a bit of experience about the loss of something we never grasped in our hands.

What dreams were lost to me? A deep-seated dream and desire of my heart was to be an organist even to owning my own pipe organ. At the time of polio our family basement was full of organ pipes and chests waiting for the time of dream fulfillment. A year after polio my organ playing dreams and my organ were lost to the reality that I would never be able to play without the use of legs and feet. The lead pipes were melted and sold as scrap; the long, bass, wooden 16' Bourdons were cut up for drawer materials. Those drawers today are a part of my shop, and do you think that each time one is opened that I do not mourn afresh? Then, of course, there was the loss of my life's dedication and dream to be a missionary and bring the gospel of Christ to those who had never heard it. Mission boards didn't want cripples. Oh, there were countless numbers of lost dreams.

These are just examples of grieving over something that we possessed only in dream form. How about grieving for those losses we actually had in our possession? My new CCM matched hockey skates were sold; my skis were sold; and my shotgun was sold. Our family was financially destitute and we knew that I would never skate, ski, or perhaps hunt again.

We certainly have as much right to grieve over both actual and dream losses, and from experience it seems to me there is little difference. If there is to be an assessment of which is the greater loss, the possession or the dream, it would seem to me that the loss of our dreams are more emotionally devastating. The *Bible* states: "*Where there is no vision* (dream) *the people perish.*" (Proverbs 29:18) Yes, the loss of a dream can be equally as crushing, and in some cases even more devastating than the loss of anything we have possessed.

At the onset of disability we do not immediately comprehend our losses. Sometimes it takes days, months, and even years for us to assess these losses. One by one they emerge from the fog, and one by one we grieve over them. With disability the grieving process is continuous as we face a deeper understanding of these new limitations.

This grieving process must take its direction and time. It usually moves in stages from denial, fantasy, reality, depression, anger or bitterness, acceptance, rehabilitation (readjusting your life), to final adjustment. It is okay for one to cry in any one of these stages. Crying washes some of the hurt away and relieves tension.

Although crying is not a problem in itself, excessive long-term crying indicates an unhealed wound. A sore, open wound invites all sorts of trouble. It is in our best interest to get it healed as rapidly as possible. But what are we talking about in terms of time? If a widow continues her deep grief and depression for much longer than one year after the loss of her husband, it is considered dangerous (and there is such a thing as dangerous grief). If you or I grieve deeply and are severely depressed for more than a year for dreams or possessions lost to disability, it is dangerous and should be treated.

This is not to say that we cannot occasionally be sad or depressed throughout our lifetime over our losses of dreams, body, or even material things. While severe grieving should be on the wane in six months, and perhaps be over in one or two years maximum, my experience has been to look at a figure of more like between three to five years of grief for an extremely traumatic loss. After the first year, however, the grief should become less intense as time heals the wound.

However, at any stage of the process, it is okay to cry—for women—and for men. It is a symptom of a deep hurt that has not yet completely healed. And we all know that even after total healing there are the scars to remind us of the hurt.

I AM NOT COURAGEOUS—I AM FRIGHTENED

Need it be said that many of my conversations in counsel with hurting people are conducted through tears. The story that follows was bathed in tears and punctuated by sobs.

> "Everyone thinks that I am so courageous to have handled John's situation so well. At our support group I overheard someone whisper, 'She is really a hero for her efforts in coping with her child's disability'. I am not a hero, not courageous, not noble, not any of those things that people say about me. Rather, I am frightened, insecure, and wounded both emotionally and spiritually.
>
> Sometimes I hate myself and sometimes I hate John, even though it was no fault of his for all this mess in our family. There are times when I want to die and times I wish John could die. No, in reality I am a terrible mother and a disgusting person."

Let me tell you about my own feelings of heroism. First of all, it was not difficult to understand this mother's horror of having heaped upon her the responsibility that accompanies heroism. Even when the deed was truly heroic, most persons shrug off the accolades and mutter, "I just did what I had to do." My insides cringe when someone refers to me as being heroic or courageous. A writer for *The St. Paul Dispatch* in St. Paul, Minnesota, back in the early seventies wrote an article about my house building skills done from a wheelchair. The reporter titled the article which appeared in the colored section of the Sunday newspaper, "The House Courage Built." It was sickening, emotional, inaccurate, and it made me nauseated.

The problem with being called courageous or heroic tends to demand that we continue to be—we are supermoms, superdads, or superBobs, and we dare not let up lest we disappoint those who believe that we are super-anything.

Let's keep in mind that all of us do things from time to time that are above and beyond the call of duty, but to expect any of us to day after day and year after year continue to impress everyone with our drive and accomplishments is foolish and destructive. One of my friends once said, "I have never heard a gripe come out of your mouth about being disabled." Not wanting to disappoint that person, my freedom of speech and expression with that person became limited.

None of us is perfect, neither should we try to be. However, when we and others expect us to be perfect, Lord, spare us from destroying ourselves by trying to meet these expectations. Remember, pedestals are great places from which to fall.

If it were my pleasure to be in a face-to-face conversation with you, and you cried, stomped the floor and said a few swear words, most likely a smile of understanding would creep over my face. You could rant and rave and you could throw up your hands in despair. You could choose to fight or surrender. However, my respect for you would not be diminished. Rather, it would be enhanced.

How well my memory brings back the picture of Supermom walking into my office and slamming the door behind her. She was the mother who did everything right for her disabled son. She was involved with United Cerebral Palsy at the local, state, and national level, and was the state area model for parents of handicapped children. She was viewed with awe by parents and professional staff alike. As the door slammed, her image crumbled as she blurted out, "I have taken this for twenty-one years, and I can't take it any longer." Alas, she was human just like we are. It was good therapy that should have taken place many years sooner. She suffered needlessly for twenty-one years with "pedestalitis." Did my impression of her devotion and her personhood diminish? No, she became a giant in my thinking.

Let none of us who is coping with disability be destroyed by people's expectations, including our own. And to the others in this world (spouse, children, friends, neighbors—yes, and even the counselors and medical practitioners), I ask simply to let us be ourselves. Allow us those times of darkness and depression. Allow us to rant and rave in honesty with our souls. Just be there to touch us and tell us that you are there if needed, and mostly that you care.

YOU CAN'T DO IT ALONE

If ever there were a person who must constantly realize that he can't do it alone, I am that person. God plopped me into this world with a insatiable drive for independence. When my mother insisted that she take me to kindergarten the first day of school, I asked her to walk far enough behind me so that the other kids would not know she was accompanying me to school. As a child I seldom asked for help on anything, but rather just struggled with it alone. And here is Mr. Independence who is forced by his disability to ask for help continuously. Even to this day, 47 years later, my inner self demands that I do it "all by myself." However, in many instances this demand cannot be met. I CANNOT do it alone.

Recently, there has been much more attention given to the needs of care givers, those devoted professionals and family members who care for those who cannot care for themselves. In the past, the emphasis was in understanding and appreciating the physical demands. Little or no thought was given to the emotional drain that accompanies giving care. With professionals it is usually 8 hours a day and 40 hours a week. With family it is sometimes 24 hours a day—7 days a week. A family caring for someone who cannot care for himself is on duty 168 hours a week and even if they sleep 8 hours each night, they are still on call. Those reading this who lack the experience and responsibility of a handicapped child, try if you can to imagine what your life would be as a mother having a sick child at home for a month—a year—a lifetime. Two weeks of chickenpox and most parents would climb the walls. You just could not do it alone.

Remember the old adage, "Many hands make light work?" Respite or relief from the demands of care giving is the only thing that will keep you sane. You may be relieved by other family members or relatives, or you might occasionally call on local groups of volunteers for your respite. Many agencies now offer respite programs that provide a few hours a day to perhaps a day a week of relief. It never ceases to amaze me how the church, with all its interest in demonstrating the love of God, does not become vibrantly active in respite care to the community. If ever there was a worthwhile service project, this is it.

Very often this care is very specialized and individual. It takes time and effort to teach other persons how to perform tasks that are essential for the care and safety of the person who is receiving this service. Because of liability and possible litigation, most respite programs only offer what could be termed as a sitting service, rejecting any "hands-on" activities. Respite care by its very nature is costly in both money and/or time. For the most difficult care situations your friends and family are your greatest asset. Unfortunately, it is often the family and close friends who would be willing to help are also the ones with whom you would like to spend your get-a-way-from-it-all time.

We also must keep in mind that many persons are not emotionally capable of dealing with disability with strangers, let alone friends. My pre-polio experiences with disabled persons were not very pleasant. After polio the reminder of disability by associating with other persons with disabilities was distasteful and I wanted to put distance between us. And then I suffered from the "guilties" for having these negative feelings. It took several years before this was conquered. Keep in mind that others do not see disability as you do. Try to remember how you reacted before you became educated by and with disability.

There always will be those who stare, some from ignorance and some from awesome compulsion. My reaction to these impolite persons is to simply ignore them. To lash out with tongue or deed at their lack of manners is to lower myself to their level. When someone inappropriately asks me why I am in a wheelchair, it is my habit to just give them the correct answer without embellishments. However, when a stranger asks me if I am capable of the sex act, I do some creative verbal conniving. One time a fellow asked me that question. My response was this: "Do you see my wife over there?"

"Yes."

"Does she have a smile on her face?

"Yes."

"Well, that's your answer.

It takes considerable time and a considerable amount of patience to educate friends, acquaintances, or volunteers in their coping with disability. Don't take it to heart if someone backs off from your request for respite. Some can handle it—some cannot; but you have no choice.

It is written in the *Bible* that *Pride cometh before the fall.* (Prov. 16:18) Your pride and mine can be our friend or our enemy. When it prevents us from asking for needed help, it is our enemy. No matter how easy or light the work, one cannot do it continuously without rest. If the care giver self destructs, who then will give the care? If you love someone enough to give them care, you also should love them enough to take care of your needs so that the care can continue.

I'LL GIVE MY LIFE

"My love is so intense that I will give up my life for that person." How many times has this reasoning come to my ears? It has been more than I care to document. So, what is wrong with parental or marital martyrdom? My child or my spouse did nothing to deserve this disability and I will give up my life so that they might live the best possible life.

Now if you are a hermit with no social entwines and having no one who gives a snap about you, your life is unencumbered like a home without a mortgage. However, if you are a part of everyday society and have someone or many who care for you or depend on you, your life is not your own with which to do selfishly as you wish. My life is no more my own than our home we live in, for it is encumbered by a mortgage and the bank has the title. Yet we say this is our home—we own it. My life and yours is encumbered by those who care about us and who lean on us for physical, emotional, spiritual, and/or financial support. My life is encumbered by a wife, two grown children, a niece, and a handful of good friends. No, my life is not totally my own to do with as I please, and most likely neither is yours.

What we are getting at here is that giving your life in service to your disabled child or spouse may be noble, but is it right or even sensible? Unfortunately, much of martyrdom has its roots in guilt and continues to be nurtured and fertilized by guilt. The guilt masks itself as love, for love is noble and guilt is sick.

The mother who has brought a disabled child into this world looks at the child and says in her heart, "It was not your fault this happened to you. My body produced you and it is my fault; therefore, I will give my life in an attempt to make up to you for failing you in development." It is extremely difficult, perhaps impossible, that a man or a father can understand the selfless devotion given to a handicapped child by a woman, especially its mother.

Unfortunately, I have seen many families destroyed by what many see as noble selflessness. There are some fathers and some families who willingly agree to this martyrdom, while others are forced to accept it. It is these forced families who self destruct. You see, you have not heard the other side of the picture from family members who were short changed by this undying devotion to a disabled family member.

There is nothing wrong with special care and love for a disabled person. It is when other persons suffer for that commitment that it becomes selfish and dangerous. Now I know that you will hear and read many stories to the contrary. What you choose to believe is your business, but it is my business to inform you that much of what has been spoken and written on this subject is lopsided and in error. No one wants to get up before a group or write an article saying that love destroyed their family, for they would be hissed. However, they say it privately to me.

Is there not a middle-of-the-road or moderate position that can be truly motivated by love rather than love/guilt? There are a few families who achieve it by not allowing the disabled person or child to be the center of the wheel on which the entire family revolves. For the disabled person's own development and benefit, he should be only a spoke in the wheel and not the center. He should be treated within his limitations the same as other family members. Within reason (and that is difficult to define) he should receive the same proportion of time as other family members.

Having been personally and professionally involved in disability for over four decades, it has been my privilege to observe and follow up on families and children involved with disability for many years, some individuals and families for as long as 40 years. Those families who have succeeded in their task of being a cohesive, successful unit are those who have adopted this middle-of-the-road philosophy. Those disabled children whom I observed over the years who became successful in entering the mainstream of life came from these homes. They were not coddled nor the center of the family wheel, just a member in good standing with all the rights and privileges of the family organization.

Family attitude toward disability is catching both within and without the family. If this chapter is pertinent to your problem, it is my suggestion that as a family you read pages 160-162 and pages 181-196 in, *"OUT OF THE ORDINARY: A Digest on Disability."*

THERE MUST BE SOMETHING I CAN DO

As a caring, devoted person we ask the question of someone with a disability, "What can I do?" Doing nothing, even when nothing can be done, flies in our face. Then we must ask, "Is it possible to do too much or do the wrong thing?"

Let's begin with the question of doing nothing when nothing apparently can be done. It is difficult for me to accept anyone's statement that there is nothing that can be done in any situation that might change the outcome. Perhaps not profoundly, but it might be changed minutely. Every person, child or adult, benefits by stimulation—stimulation to look, read, move, think, or whatever. In the case of disability the goal should be to stimulate the area of defectiveness. Physical and occupational therapists can suggest many exercises and activities for proper stimulation. Do what you can in that area, but don't make it an obsession.

Can we do the wrong thing? One of the great damaging effects is making any person, disabled or not, the center of the family attention and activity. In times long past, this was called "spoiling" the child (or even an adult). It would not be in good sense or taste to involve ourselves at this point in the great controversial philosophies of discipline. The biblical injunction is adaptable to any philosophy: *"He that spares the rod hates his son, but he who loves him is diligent to discipline him."* (Proverbs 13:24) Don't be misled by the term rod. In the *Bible* as in Psalm 23, the rod was an instrument that was used to guide sheep, not to beat them.

It is very easy to overlook a child's social development when a disability is present. One mother said to me, "How can I or anyone discipline a handicapped child? Haven't they been treated badly enough by life? How can anyone deny them anything they want?"

The current theme in discipline is "Tough Love." Tough love is tougher on parents than on the child. It is much easier to give in and say yes when we know the answer should be an emphatic NO. If you don't discipline your child with love—tough love—society in time will discipline with dislike, disgust, and probable rejection. Which do you prefer?

In our family we had the true story of the mother bear. When our kids were 8 and 12 years of age, our extended family had a cabin near Finland, Minnesota, up near the North Shore of Lake Superior. We often went to the refuse dump hoping to see the bears. One year the local high point was a mother bear with twin cubs. We were rewarded with their presence and we watched intently as they rummaged through the garbage. Suddenly, the mother bear gave out a strange grunt. One cub scampered up a tree while the other remained an instant longer to finish off his morsel. Wham! The mother cuffed the cub and sent him sprawling.

"What a mean mother," our kids said almost in unison. Then we explained (not in these words) that the purpose of parenting was to ready the off-spring for independence in the world, should it live so long. The cuff might very well save the cub's life in a more real life-or-death situation. The kids nodded in understanding, and later when discipline was administered, all we had to say was, "Remember the mother bear?"

Our responsibility as parents is to prepare our children, disabled or not, for the world to come. How well we succeed in this will determine much of their success in life. It is the rule and not the exception that parents of disabled children will focus their efforts on the medical aspects of the disability. They leave no stones unturned in a search for doctors, clinics, or therapeutic methods that offer a shred of hope in helping to correct the disability.

While this medical obsession is in force, all too often the social development of the child is ignored or left to chance. You feel that if you can just get this messed up body straightened out, everything else will fall into place.

Sorry, but this is not the case. In my work with adults who were born with or who acquired their disabilities in early childhood, in many cases these persons were physically able to perform in our programs. But alas, the behavioral problems encountered in those whose discipline and social development had been neglected, were so glaring that we were forced to drop them from the program. Parents were stunned. Ask any person with long-term experience in working with the disabled which is more important, a good body or a good social development. Ask me. My answer would be that there is more hope for a person with a severely limited mind or body than one with severe behavioral difficulties.

Many of you are familiar with the story of Bree Walker, the beautiful, successful TV news anchorwoman who has ectrodactylism (split hand or split foot syndrome). Although her feet are apparently normal, she has what amounts to clubs for hands. It is a genetic disorder, her mother and one brother being similarly challenged. In one interview she stated how important it was for her that her parents insisted that her disability not be used as an excuse to get out of doing things or allow her to wallow in self pity. This helped her develop a good self image.

The problem is that love is blind—not only romantic love but family love as well. Parents are often blind to the social "sins" of their children. All that we can ask of you is that you give the same benefits of social development to your handicapped child as you do your other children. In my mind to do less is criminal. That is bitter language, but I can find no way to sweeten it.

Looking From Inside Out

This final segment on counsel to parents with handicapped children is best written by Ruth Gullerud. By way of introduction, Ruth has the distinction of being very limited by cerebral palsy at birth, struggling through those early years of childhood, adolescence, and finally adulthood. She was another of those persons who adjusted well to life and to her disability because her parents saw no reason to treat her differently than any other child—tough love.

She has the advantage of speaking from a standpoint of being "the handicapped child," as well as from the position of being professionally involved with adults and children with disabilities. She has a graduate counseling degree and has been a counselor with United Cerebral Palsy of West Central Wisconsin for 16 years, and their very-successful Executive Director for the past 12 years.

Parenting Skills: More Alike Than Different

by Ruth Gullerud

Parents often ask me to describe the greatest factors occurring in my childhood which assured my success as an adult. The answer is a puzzle to me and not one readily apparent. But I suspect that the key has something to do with growing up in the wake of losing my mother at birth, being expected to reach the highest possible achievements, and struggling to be educated by normal standards in pre-mainstreamed school days.

I also believe there were other influences of more tangible impact, ones that any parent needs to ponder. I especially remember how my screaming and kicking tantrums were chastened with spankings and lengthy periods of sitting in the corner to contemplate the rewards of such unacceptable behavior. Grandma, my childhood guardian and friend, left no room for my doubting that any rules passed down from six other brothers and sisters were to apply equally to me. My butt and pride still sting from such recollections, but self-expectations of equal social performance were established early and continue to prevail.

I recall, with beads of sweat on my brow, how my father and grandmother would station themselves on opposite ends of the carpet, encouraging me to crawl, and later walk, between them. The distance, which now measured a few feet, then stretched into horrendous and tearful laps. But I always knew that the rewards of comforting hugs would come only if I tried and my performance measured up to the average of the week before.

"Never say can't before you try, and always measure your best by your own record of performance." And with that advice I eventually moved into pursuing college, ignoring professional skepticism, and later into reaching vocational status realized by my own achievable goals.

Today, having spent several years tracing the same paths with other families experiencing the challenges of a child with a disability, I do have some observations to offer. Most importantly, please realize that they are the ones applied to the careful caring of *any* child, challenged by disability or simply by growing up.

A frequent occurrence in families rearing children having severe disabilities is that the immense attention required to address physical needs has caused critical neglect of the discouragement of unacceptable behavior. Counselors working with disabled adults frequently wish they could have impacted on the early development of their clients. An individual who has achieved independent walking but who has not learned to respect the needs of others will, without fail, meet with less success than that wheelchair user who listens and shares.

Remembering specific individuals I have counseled who have exhibited critical delays in social skills, several common concerns recur. The disabled adult who is meeting negative self-image very often displays self-defeating traits:

- Reluctance to share.
- Inability to stop self-focusing and to listen.
- Neglecting to express thanks.
- Difficulty in finding ways to return favors and in recognizing the need to do so.
- Ignoring the value of maintaining personal appearance (e.g. cleaning wheelchair, laundering clothes).

In the same spirit as dreaming that your small child will become a prosperous citizen, do your handicapped child the following lifelong favors:

- Dare to establish consistent rules, enforced with loving discipline.
- Insist on acceptable social skills (good manners, sharing, respecting others).
- Encourage independence to every extent reasonable.
- Help to identify acceptable expressions of frustrations (which surely will come).
- Assign responsibilities to whatever ability level is achievable.

Admittedly, the toughest assignment to effective parenting a disabled child is going to be the subduing of your own grief, your feelings of sympathy for your child's "unfortunate" condition. Once you have overcome that hurdle, you will see that your child is just as naughty and as challenging of your patience as the other children in the neighborhood. And you will be able to view your child headed toward adulthood and be able to lovingly provide the tools necessary for a happy integration with society.

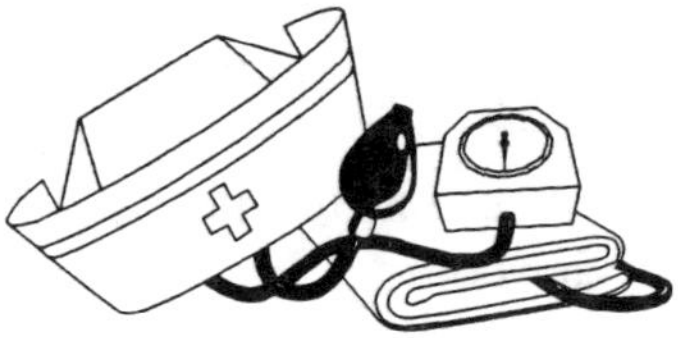

Chapter 3

FAMILY AND FRIENDS

HANDS-ON CARE
GIVEN BY SPOUSE OR FAMILY MEMBER

Before we begin let's define terms. Spouse is much more easily defined than care giver. Spouse is husband or wife, but what is a care giver? Although my spouse assists me with some tasks that I cannot do for myself or those that are extremely taxing, she does not consider herself a care giver in the usual sense. The term lends itself easily to have the connotation of physical nursing care: toileting, bathing, feeding, dressing, getting the person with a disability out of bed and ready for the day, and any number of tasks that require a great amount of time and effort. For those of us who simply need a few physical assists with difficult or impossible small tasks, care giver gives the wrong impression.

Sometimes it is a brother, sister or friend who has become involved in giving care. If your lives are entwined physically or financially, you tend to fit the spouse model. So for those of you who are care givers who are not the spouse but in a sense fit these circumstances, please fill in your name mentally when I have written spouse.

For those newly-disabled persons who have just come home from the hospital or rehabilitation center, very often the spouse and/or care giver steps in for a brief or long-term commitment of truly giving care. The duration and degree of assistance depend on the success of the disabled person's rehabilitation in all aspects of life. In the first months after polio, I needed care. As I learned to do things for myself, that care was reduced to zero within four months.

Nonetheless, it is a rude awakening for a family when reality begins to sink in that a functioning member has become limited and is unable to do today what that person could do a week, a month, or a year ago. It may take months to years to determine the extent of these limitations and how it will ultimately affect all those concerned. There are often long hospital stays with even longer periods of rehabilitation.

Along this route your family cries out for information on what to expect and what to do. At first these are simple questions:

1. Is my wife or husband going to live?
2. How long is the treatment going to be necessary?
3. When can I bring them home?
4. Will insurance cover these costs?

Let's take a brief look at each of these four questions and later an additional four. The question of life/death is usually answered within a few days to a few weeks. If death was the result you would most likely not be reading this book. It is life, then, that confronts us. Unfortunately, there are times in which modern medical technology does us no favors with its life-saving techniques and support systems. So often the medical community breaks its arm patting itself on the back for saving and sustaining a life, only to relegate that "saved" person, and often a family, to a life of misery.

Too often my experience with disability has revealed the absolute hell that sometimes accompanies the saving of a life rather than the joy that would be expected. Don't be fooled. Too many medical personnel feel it is their duty to only walk you and your spouse to the door of the medical facility, certainly not out into the main street of reality of the remainder of this person's newly-limited life. The diagnosis and treatment is the end of their responsibility and now it is up to the family, and the person himself. Often there is no referral to any person or agency to help this family. I am sure there is concern, but it is not reflected in any non-medical advice or other direction.

One time at a professional rehabilitation meeting I made the mistake of expressing my mind. One of the counselors was describing his client and saying there was nothing that could be done. My comment on hearing the extensive and severe limitations that an accident had placed on this young man was that it was too bad that he had lived. Those within earshot of my statement were aghast at my attitude and challenged me with angry looks and angry words. "Who are you to play God?," one counselor snorted.

My reply was simple and terse. "I am not playing God, simply offering my opinion, and it appears that you all disagree with me which is your privilege. But let me remind you that you are all walking around as reasonably-normal persons and that none of you has experienced the physical and emotional agony of a disability. So my suggestion to you is that until you have had personal experience with either yourself or someone in your family who has become severely limited in body or mind, you temper your criticisms of those who have had the experience." Then there was deathly silence.

There are also questions regarding the other aspects of disability that are related to the medical treatment of your spouse. More often than not, this treatment period will last longer and cost more than you ever dreamed. At age eighteen when I contracted polio, it was assumed by our family and me that it would be perhaps only several weeks and it would all be completed—I would be back at home, work, and school in just a matter of a few weeks.

Well, it was not a few weeks; it was thirteen months in the hospital and another year of outpatient therapy. It was two years, not two months. The results—I left the medical facility as a paraplegic with no hope of any improvement. No, this was not the end of my life, but only its beginning. Was I discouraged? No, and I don't want you to be either. In a later segment it is my hope that the shared experiences of mine and other's will help give motivation to look at your situation with challenge rather than despair.

MONEY! MONEY! MONEY!

Money! Our lives revolve around money, so it is not unusual that one of your first questions will be related to costs. As you are aware, medical costs for any type of treatment are astronomical. Most families are not prepared for the financial shock of these costs. In today's world you must be either very rich or very poor to have medical expenses related to long-term therapy or extended hospital stays satisfied that are not covered by medical insurance. Most of us are neither very rich nor very poor, so that means we are discussing the problems of Mr. Average and Mrs. Middleclass. Without good and continued medical insurance coverage or large personal resources, you are faced with an either/or situation. You either go without those medical or therapeutic services or you suffer the possibilities of financial ruin.

Guilt keeps all of us from making wise decisions in this either/or situation. You want to do everything that is humanly possible for your spouse or loved one. And as I sit here thinking about what I would do for my wife regarding any need she might have, my heart says that I would spend my last dime and go to the limit of debt for her. But is that what she would want? I asked her and she answered an emphatic NO. Then she asked, "Do you want me to spend our last dime on your care?" Of course not, but we know if we didn't that we might suffer eternal guilt feelings.

My experience on this issue is that you are better off limiting the treatment than subjecting yourself and/or spouse as well as the family to the trauma of possible bankruptcy. If you self-destruct financially, physically, or emotionally, who and what is left for care of that person you love?

Sometimes we do our biggest favor to those we love by not doing them a favor. No one can tell you what services you should have for your spouse or loved one or what your financial limits should be. However, be aware of the fact that emotions destroy whatever good financial sense you might have had before you were faced with this problem.

Home Sweet Home

And finally, out of the hospital or rehabilitation center back home. Home! What a beautiful word. The wall hanging, "Home, Sweet Home," now has new meaning to both you and your loved one. As I lay in my hospital bed unable to move, my mind told me that if somehow I could just get home things would be normal again, but it turned out to be anything but normal. My first visit home was nearly three months after polio struck and my sitting-up time had just been extended to thirty minutes a day. Just getting me into the car to drive me home for a few hours was an ordeal.

The steps into the house that had presented no problem just a few months ago were now insurmountable. Because my father had been sidelined with heart disease and a recent stroke, our family arranged for a neighbor to carry me into the house and lay me on the couch.

What about the bathroom? I knew that if nature called it was going to be big trouble. But I was home and it was wonderful for those few hours even with all the problems. Our naiveté prevented us from anticipating all the thorns that presented themselves in the rose of those early home visits.

You must be alert to the possibility of much the same experience. Although the home is the same as when your loved one left, very possibly neither they nor you are the same as in the past. Your lifestyle has perhaps changed forever, and you are playing a new game with new rules. Much of your success in playing this new game rests upon your shoulders, and much of the success of your loved one's playing this new game rests upon him/her. Let's get one thing straight right here: you each bear equal responsibility in making a new life for yourselves, one that includes the limitations imposed on your loved one.

The preceding paragraphs have been directed to those situations in which there was some catastrophic happening—a stoke, an injury accident, or something that changed overnight. How about the spouse who has a terminal illness or otherwise progressively-worsening disorder? Your life undergoes radical change, but over a longer period of time. There are some advantages to this in that you have more time to adjust and develop a new perspective. If you are wise, you will see this as an opportunity for good long-term planning in finances, modifications to home, family planning, employment, long-term care, and in many other areas. If you are wise you will use this time to your best advantage rather than put your head in the sand and hope your troubles will blow away. They won't, and you will find yourself engulfed in panic situations.

There are two prefixes to thought—fore(thought) and after(thought). Your own experiences in life so far should have taught you the sometimes-disastrous costs of afterthought. Don't be its victim, for it is costly in all the areas of concern to you at the moment—financial, emotional, and physical.

As you find answers to the first group of questions, they are replaced by these:

1. Will my spouse be able to return to work?
2. Is there pain with this condition or disease?
3. What won't my spouse be able to do that was done before?
4. What can I expect next month or next year?

In a world where we seem to have answers for just about everything, it comes as a shock when you ask these questions and we just can't seem to get answers. The problem is that at the time the answers to these questions are most needed, they are the least available. Much of the time this is because there are no accurate answers during this crucial first year after an accident, disease, or condition has been injected into your life.

Most of today's households seem to require both husband and wife to work. Whether this is a necessity or simply the desire to have more for you and your family is not a part of the question. The question is this, "If my spouse cannot return to work, what will we do?" Most of us do not like the obvious answer, and that is to lower our standard of living to balance with our reduced income. We plead, "My kids will have to forego a college education; we will have to sell our home; there will be no travel vacations, etc."

We are perhaps correct, but we have the option of balancing our budget now or destroying ourselves financially a few miles down the road. I have seen more than one family who has lost its home and are in financial ruin because they refused to believe that in the United States there was any other way to go than UP. They could not or would not accept the fact that they got a lousy deal from life and it was going to require sacrifices by every family member. I would like to take the time and space to tell you how to avoid this pitfall, but if my forewarning is not sufficient to put you on alert and have you enact some changes, my solutions would also be useless.

From my vantage point of over sixty-five years of living life, forty-seven of these in a wheelchair and forty as a counselor, let me assure you that a college education is not necessarily a ticket to vocational or financial success. Furthermore, it is not necessary to attend the finest universities, but it is necessary for your children to extract the most learning from their educations and to get the highest grades possible. Any person over the age of eighteen can attend a community college and be employed at the same time. For the gifted student there is always the grant or scholarship. In today's field of education, lack of funds is no excuse for not graduating from college; the only valid excuses are lack of motivation and lack of ability.

There are no psychological or sociological studies that prove that a child without his own bedroom or bathroom is destined to mediocrity.

The only deprivation that destroys a child is the deprivation of love, not things. Designer clothes haven't added one point to a child's IQ or $10 a month to his earning power. Being poor is no sin. My experience in my own life and eight years of post-high school education is that those who struggled the most gained the most from their education—no pain, no gain.

Our problem is that those of us who grew up during the Great Depression don't want our own kids to want for anything. To me, that is the greatest fallacy of our generation. We have the potential for destroying the very persons we love by indulging them. If you feel guilty about having to cut back on the goodies or even the basics because of your loved one's disability, just keep in mind that the family that struggles together survives together.

On to the subject of pain. Of course there is pain with every disability, some of it is physical and some of it is emotional. Experience in life has most likely taught you that emotional pain is more difficult to cope with than is physical pain. The problem with disability is that the entire family suffers from emotional pain, but your spouse most likely suffers from both.

Every person has a different tolerance for either emotional pain or physical pain. You must also come to grips with your own and your spouse's limitations in coping with it. In a counseling session the wife looked at me tearfully and said, "It hurts me deeply to see my husband out in the yard hanging up the wash; that's my job and it makes me feel useless and unneeded." That was a pain that aspirin could not touch, and there are many others.

Even though the mind thinks in terms of wholeness, the body cannot cooperate and perform many of those tasks that were so effortless in times past. It is difficult for the newly-disabled person and the family to realize just how limiting a disability can be.

How about food preparation and cooking? The kitchen is a disaster area for working from a wheelchair with its high counters and no leg/foot room. All tasks must be done sitting sidesaddle and twisting ninety degrees. Try peeling a potato with one hand. Try it yourself to get a feel for all these things that your now-limited loved one is forced to do. Spend a day in a wheelchair, or tie one arm to your waist, or in bed with your hands tied at your side and having to ask for assistance to turn over, eat, drink, swat a fly on your face, pee, or you-name-it.

Two words adequately describe this experience—humiliation and frustration. In your position as care giver, you only have to deal with frustration, not humiliation. Please don't get the impression that I am on your back. It is a two-way street.

There are two types of loss to consider: 1) loss of what your spouse can no longer do for you, and 2) loss of what your spouse can no longer do for him or herself. All too often when someone becomes disabled to the point of needing assistance in what we commonly call Activities of Daily Living (ADL), those who must do those tasks for them find themselves in a unique and frustrating position. Most often the "doee" is not happy about needing this care, and the "doer" is unhappy about having to perform the care.

It is not a happy situation no matter how we look at it. However, both your attitude as well as your loved one's toward the demands of this care will not necessarily make it a happy one, but it can certainly add some pleasant aspects and make it a little brighter if you will let it.

Frayed Emotions

It is important for you to understand some of the surprising behavior that will no doubt be observed by the recipient of your care and you toward each other. It is not uncommon for persons who are hurting to lash out at the one they love most. Some of you may remember The Ink Spots' recording of this song:

> "You always hurt the one you love, the one you shouldn't hurt at all.
> You always take the sweetest rose and crush it 'til the petals fall.
> You always break the kindest heart with a hasty word you can't recall.
> So if I broke your heart last night, its because I love you most of all."

Hurting one you love is a conundrum, but both you and I know how true it is. Sometimes the person receiving the care lashes out in anger, not at you personally, but what you represent—you and your care become a symbol of what they can no longer do for themselves, and so they strike out at you. This is unfair but understandable. This anger can only be directed at two things, people or objects. I have seen persons under the influence of frustration throw grape jelly on the family's new drapes, or to strike an emotional blow with words from the mouth when it was the only part that had no limitation.

Many years ago a couple came to me with their troubles. He was a quadriplegic with practically no use of his arms and hands. She was an occupational therapist who met him in a hospital and they had married. At that time they had one child and their relationship was beginning to sour. All she did was to wait on him and their child and she was getting tired of those demands. On one occasion he was full of lip and chastised her verbally for some minor infraction, and then managed with his limited swing to push the jelly sandwich she was eating in her face. In retaliation she grabbed the full pitcher of Kool Aid and poured it over his head. And now this couple who had tried so hard to cope with disability were in my office seeking counsel.

When I heard their story I committed the unpardonable sin. I tried so hard but could not contain my laughter and I let out a rocking guffaw. As I came "unglued," they in turn looked at each other and began to laugh.

Then we discussed the problems of care giving as we are in this book, and they saw they were not mean, ugly people, but persons who were responding in a very normal way to a very abnormal situation. A week later she called to tell me how much help their session had been and that they had canceled their appointment with a psychiatrist whom they had been seeing prior to our visit.

However, you must understand that just because something is normal, it is not necessarily correct. Had that behavior continued it would have been the end of their relationship. As you develop an understanding for your unusual behavior, you will also find that it changes. Damaging behavior exposed to the truth should not remain unchanged. If snakes are coming into your house through a hole in the foundation, who in his right mind would not upon discovery plug the hole?

In the Summer 1992 issue of *ACCENT on living* magazine, an excellent example of frayed emotions can be found in which the editor requested solutions from the readers of how they might have solved Shelli's burn-out problem from giving care. Her article is reprinted by permission in Chapter 7, MARRIED COUPLES.

Oh, For The Crystal Ball

Finally, what does the future hold? Oh, for the proverbial crystal ball. There are many months and years of adjustment ahead. Know that both you and your spouse will go through the usual stages of mourning a loss, for you both lost some things very dear to you. Keep in mind that your losses are equally as painful even though they are not identical. Being uniquely human, there are no two persons who will experience identical mourning periods. Neither are there any two persons with identical disabilities, identical personalities, or identical futures. Even though no one can predict your spouse's or your future, you and he or she do have more control over it than you might feel you do.

You do have some control of your attitudes toward each other and toward the disability itself. These attitudes have a great effect on you individually as well as your future together. Negative feelings toward each other or toward the disability itself can only produce a negative outcome. Positive feelings can only produce a positive outcome. If this loved one is your spouse, don't either of you hold your mate hostage to what happened, for neither of you are happy about the whole thing. Hostage holding is when a spouse holds the other responsible in some way for the disability and makes demands for ransom. In a great sense, your future together is what you make it. Isn't that the same as the day you walked down the aisle together and said your vows?—that your future depended upon strong efforts from both of you?

For The Family: Mothers, Fathers, Sisters, And Brothers

Make no mistake, disability is a family affair. Disability has its effect on every person who has any love for the person who has become limited by a disability, and that includes friends, both the family friends and the friends of the person with the disability. In this segment we will discuss only the immediate family and we will discuss friends later. Keep in mind that a husband/wife relationship is not the same as father-mother-sisters-brothers. Marriage implies unity and duty.

Let's begin with mother. You carried this child for approximately nine months; you put your life on the line in the delivery room; you fed, clothed, bathed, protected this child; you directed this child until he or she graduated to adulthood and no longer needed or wanted your instinctive services. That is the natural order of nature—prepare your offspring for an independent life. However, in the human species we do not turn our backs on our offspring after they are weaned. With us humans it is "once a parent, always a parent." Most mothers would give their lives for their child at any age. It makes no difference if our children are two, twenty, forty, or sixty, they are yet our children and we never lose that feeling of protective, parental behavior. Disability is a family affair.

How about father? I am a father and I also had a father with whom I was very close. When my son was a year old he was playing outside in his playpen. My dad and I were visiting by the playpen when he stared at me for a few seconds, then at the ground, and uttered, "How would you feel if when he (my son) got to be eighteen he was paralyzed for the rest of his life?" As he looked up at me there were tears rolling down his wrinkled cheeks. That's all he ever said about his reaction to my contracting polio, but I never forgot those tears and the look on his face. Seventeen years after his death when my son became eighteen, at least a partial understanding of my father's emotions became real as I looked at this big 6'1" healthy, walking kid of ours and relived my polio experience, but with me as the father and him as the victim. Disability is a family affair.

And then there are sisters. My oldest sister was more like a mother to me than a sister. My middle sister married and left home before I was four so I never really knew her as a sister, but nonetheless I was her little brother. I was the last of three and we were far enough apart so that there was no sibling rivalry. It is a general rule that brothers are special to sisters as are fathers to daughters; and sisters are special to brothers as mothers are to sons. Don't wonder why you hurt so much when disaster befalls your sister or brother. You will cry and grieve like your parents are doing, but it will be from a different perspective. Disability is a family affair.

Do grandma and grandpa care about what happened? Yes, and they grieve on par with the parents and siblings. Coming late in my parent's life, I only knew one grandparent and I always assumed that she had so many grandchildren it was not much of a hurt to her that I was now paralyzed. Wrong! This old lady had suffered heartaches all of her life and she had never had "the good life." She was born just after the Civil War in the then rough-and-tumble new state of Minnesota. She had lost triplets shortly after birth, a twin grandchild at age two, and a grandson from a stray bullet. She was a stoic Englishwoman who never showed emotion. Simply because a family member does not openly or outwardly express hurt, that is no indication that it is non-existent. I am sure grandma cried for me, herself and for her son and family who were going through this terrible ordeal. Disability is a family affair.

It has only been recently that I have become aware of how each family member had been affected by my disability. My sister, who had been writing family history said to me, "I have always wanted to tell my side of your polio experience." Therefore, one of her stories was about how she and the other family members reacted to my contracting polio. My mother was nearly devastated by my paralysis, but it was now over forty years later that I began to realize what my polio had done to her. She did a lot of crying that was never known to me. After all, I was the one who was paralyzed; shouldn't I be the one to grieve if there was to be any?

I had picked up my father and brought him home from the hospital two days before the first symptoms of polio were apparent in me. He had suffered a blood clot to the brain and could not drive or work, or think and talk straight. Several weeks later he sat at the dining room table and sobbed when he could not compose a letter to me in the hospital.

My oldest sister followed the ambulance to the hospital to admit me, and no family member saw me again for nearly three weeks because of strict isolation from the polio virus. She wrote that she managed to keep from emotional collapse on her way to the hospital because she knew she had to be emotionally stable to be able to complete the registration.

My middle sister flew from Washington, D.C., as soon as I was out of isolation and could see people. This family cried together, they prayed together, and they grieved together. Disability is a family affair.

As our family attempted to put their emotional lives back together, it was obvious that their intent also was to help me recover emotionally, physically, and spiritually to the highest level possible. Our family had no money, and financial help was not possible. However, our family did have one great asset, and that was sticking together in times of trouble, and this was one of those times. They were encouraging within the realm of reason; they did whatever they could to get me pointed in the right direction again, just as they had done in my childhood and early teens. They let me know in deeds that they were around for me to *use* as I attempted to remake my new life in a wheelchair.

Notice, please, in that last sentence the word use. There are more appropriate words, but USE was chosen for a reason. Persons with a disability need to use those family members around them in their struggle for rehabilitation. There is nothing wrong with using or borrowing another person's limbs or skills. The problems arise when we *AB-use* these benefits. Abraham Lincoln was reported to have stated: "You do not help a man if you do something for him that he can do for himself."

Family, scratch that indelibly on every wall of your home. The greatest hindrance to recovery is for someone to do for us what we can (and should) do for ourselves. The problem comes in learning what a person with a disability can and cannot do for himself. In the early stages of rehabilitation no one really knows his capabilities of that moment—not the person with the disability, his parents, his family, his friends, or the medical practitioners. However, when you are sure that your family member can do it, even with much difficulty, don't let them do it, MAKE them do it for their own good.

In those early days when I had the privilege of leaving the hospital and visiting home on Sundays, there were three-plus persons standing by me to do my bidding. One of those times I dropped a pencil on the floor and three people made a dive for it. However, before they managed to get their hands on it and give it to me, the family was brought to attention by my yowl. "Please don't do this to me. Let me try and get it myself no matter how much I must struggle. When I finally give up I will ask for help." That's how the pencil episode ended and it was the family rule for a lifetime. Can you understand how important it is to be available for help that is necessary, but unavailable for help that is not absolutely necessary?

Do you practice what you preach, Buster? No, I do not do every little thing for myself that is possible. As a half person in a whole world I have competed in every way. However, without some of those little things that my wife, and sometimes my children and friends do for me, my life would be even more frustrating and fatiguing. If I transfer to my recliner and forget to bring the TV remote with me, it is very kind of someone to bring it to me when they have a few seconds. For me to get in and out of that recliner is a project in and of itself, so the best approach is to remember the dang thing in the first place.

Demands for time and demands for service by a person limited by a disability need to be rationed on a priority basis. All too often, a person with these limitations gets the notion that it is his right to demand service. Part of the great manipulation of persons with disabilities is to make the family feel guilty if they don't bow to servanthood. When asked to do a task that makes you grit your teeth and growl silently, it is time for some good old-fashioned conversation. It is better for everyone if you are honest with each other, even when you think it might hurt—and most often it does. Stick to your guns, family, but clear the air with as much open conversation of the facts and feeling of the situation as possible.

As brothers and sisters, keep in mind that serving your disabled sibling should be looked at and treated as a gift, not a duty. Unless you are a paid attendant, you owe that family person with a disability absolutely nothing. If you feel abused or put upon, or you assume the role of servant, it is because you chose it and/or accepted it. You have a non-binding contract which you are free to break at your pleasure. It should be your goal to help because you want to help, not because you have to help. It should be motivated by love and not duty. Have I made my point, that disability is a family affair?

For Friends And Relatives

It is common in our family to quote the oft-spoken truism: you can choose your friends, but you cannot choose your relatives. However, from your relatives oftentimes come deep and lasting friendships with aunts, uncles, cousins, in-laws, etc. We are not going to spend any time discussing relationships with relatives who are not friends; therefore, in that sense we are talking about friends, some who may happen to be relatives, and the same feelings and rules of friendship apply.

Man is a social being and craves interaction with other like beings. As one gains experience in life, it becomes evident that good, close friends are like cultured pearls. They are a beautiful and costly product of man and nature in cooperation with each other. As do these pearls, friends need time and cultivation to enhance their value. One day my wife and I, along with some close friends of ours, were trying to decide some test of good friendship. Somehow we came to the conclusion that a good test would be if you called a friend, asked to borrow $1,000 immediately, with no questions asked, no signed note, and no agreement on payback, that a good friend would loan you the money if he had it. Not too many of us have such friends, but most of us have someone to whom we can turn in times of trouble as well as share our joy. These relationships we all have vary in intensity of cohesiveness, and range from the $1,000-loan persons down to mere acquaintances.

Friendships usually begin with some mutual interest and develop into respect and admiration over a period of time. When my son was twelve years of age he returned from a Scouting event. I noticed that he seemed to be depressed. I asked him what was bothering him and he replied, "Nothing." Two more days of gloom and I pinned him down saying that there was something bothering him and I wanted to know what it was. Then it came tumbling out: "Daddy, did you ever like someone real much at first, and then when you got to know them better you didn't like them very much at all?" I nodded my head and told him that had happened to me many times—and continues to happen.

We talked about friends and how important they are to us, and sometimes the opposite happened, that we might not like someone at first, and then as we became better acquainted, we liked them very much. Over and over these friendships are tested through the years. Some survive; others don't.

Some friendships are based on what your friend can do for you; some are based on what your friend can do with you; while others are based on mutual love and respect. Now on the line is the most crucial of all tests of friendships, your friend becomes disabled in some way.

If your friendship was based primarily on what that person could do for you and you no longer can get a payoff from that friend, goodbye friend. If your relationship was built primarily on some mutual enjoyment in which your newly-disabled friend can no longer participate—sports, camping, hobbies, etc.—goodbye friend. Now we are down to those friendships that are primarily based on love, respect, and just having a good time together no matter what you are doing. Very often these relationships last a lifetime and become one of our most precious possessions—like the pearls cultured by time and love. It is not my intention to leave you with the idea that I think in pure black/white terms of friendship. Most friendships contain varying amounts of "do for," "do with," and "mutual closeness."

Suddenly, and perhaps without warning your friend is found face to face with adversity—some type of physical, emotional, or intellectual limitation. It may have been an auto or industrial accident; it may have been a newly-diagnosed disease or condition; or it may be a terminal illness. The friend may improve, perhaps stabilize, become progressively worse, or may die. You know not which of these it will be.

Your relationship can no longer be the same as it was. It may be closer; it may be more distant; but it cannot be the same—believe me. Your mind is in turmoil. What can you do? First and foremost you can be honest—honest with yourself and honest with your friend in every situation. At first you will both be walking a tightrope in this new aspect of your friendship. Leave out the nitpicky stuff, but when something major bugs you about your friend, you must inform your now-disabled friend of this diplomatically and honestly. And if you can't do it diplomatically, you at least can do it honestly. Unfortunately, the art of diplomacy is a lost cause with some persons. You, your friend, or both of you may be one of these persons.

Pity is the one ingredient that I do not need, nor does any other person who is disabled. There is a fine line between pity and empathy and there is a certain amount of interchange with these two emotions. Pity: "Sympathetic grief or sorrow, excited by the suffering or misfortune of another, often leading one to give aid or to show mercy." Empathy: "Intellectual identification with, or vicarious experiencing of the feelings, thoughts, or attitudes of another person." Which of these definitions is the motivating force in your desire to help your friend? I have never asked for nor wanted pity; but I do desire understanding from the world, my neighbors, my friends, relatives, and my wife and children.

Your behavior at this time is an indicator of the type and intensity of your friendship. There is nothing wrong with having "do for" and "do-with" friends, so don't develop a case of the "guilties" if your interest soon fades. However, you may have been surprised by your own grief and concern for your friend. Perhaps this experience has caused you to re-evaluate your relationship and you find it deeper than you realized. Know that if you continue your relationship, you will suffer some emotional wounds. If there ever was a time your friend needed you, it is now, whether you are a former co-worker, neighbor, childhood or school chum, relative, or whatever.

What you must learn as quickly as possible is that unless your friend had brain damage he or she is the same person. They may behave differently; they may be angry and abusive to you; they may turn their back on you for a time. This emotional and physical turmoil they are enduring is the ultimate test of character and personality. You have no idea how you or anyone else would react under similar circumstances. Each of us reacts uniquely to a disability or emotional trauma.

Suddenly you find yourself absorbed in your friend's troubles. Sometimes you laugh with them; sometimes you cry with them. They make demands on your time and energies. Sometimes you might find yourself being the advocate or go-between in families, medical facilities, and health agencies. Friendship cannot be a one-way street. You must receive something in return. It may be just the feeling of deep satisfaction of helping someone. It may be that you did have a good time just being together as in times past. However, both you and your friend must keep in mind that friendship is a mutual giving and receiving.

Again I warn you not to destroy your friend by allowing them to become dependent upon you. Your goal should be to help them help themselves. Don't let yourself be trapped in a rut; for example, do not take your friend shopping or engage in any other activity on an absolute, regular schedule. This friend must learn how to function without you. That means finding alternatives to grocery shopping (or whatever) on occasion. Do you have any idea what happens to your friend if you do not help them develop independence? For whatever reason, when you cannot do or continue to perform these services (even just an afternoon or evening visit), your friend is doomed. Alas, they have no alternative sources.

The two greatest enemies of persons with disabilities are idleness and isolation. You can be a part of the vital solution to these enemies. Involve your friend in a project; give them some responsibility and something to do. Go out into the community and do things together. Of course you will receive some stares and at times be confronted with problems for which the only solution is to go home. You must learn your friend's limitations and often scout out a restaurant or facility to see if it is accessible for your friend.

The wheelchair accessibility symbol is world-wide, and it is to inform you that a facility is accessible. Unfortunately, these symbols sometimes "lie," and you cannot count on them. I have seen the symbol on rest room doors through which a wheelchair could not even pass through the entrance door, say nothing of the many in which the toilet stalls, washbowls, and towels were inaccessible. Some establishments think that installing a grab bar in a toilet stall makes the rest room accessible.

For a successful day or night on the town, learn to be a good scout. Do it ahead of time. Call the restaurant for reservations and ask about accessibility and their ability to handle your friend. What your friend doesn't need is the sour experience of being a spectacle and being humiliated in front of a host of people. I can tell you from my own experience and those experiences related to me by hundreds of others, that we would rather stay home than to suffer from these humiliations. Learning the importance of scouting out the problems and solving them before they happen comes with experience. If you will learn it now, it will save you untold unhappy situations with your friend.

On two occasions I have held up the departure of an airliner for thirty minutes. Why? They didn't have the equipment readily available to load me. I was finally carried onto the plane and dumped awkwardly into a seat while the entire crew and passengers gawked—so this was the guy who was holding up takeoff. It was not my idea of fun, and I have very tough emotional skin for things of this nature.

If you anticipate a long-lasting relationship with your friend, consider their needs if you build a new home or rent a new apartment. If I can't get up your steps it is obvious there can be no visit. If I can't get into your bathroom it should also be quite obvious that my visit will of necessity be short. Portable aluminum ramps can be purchased to make a trip up one-to-four steps as safe as possible. Furniture can be rearranged, and sometimes doors can be rehung. In a later segment I will get into the specifics of wheelchair accessibility for those interested.

It is my opinion that there is no able-bodied person who can possibly comprehend the put-down that an architectural barrier is to those of us who have a disability in which that barrier prevents or makes difficult our independent functioning. It is like throwing water in our faces as the ultimate slam. There is no greater reminder of our disabilities than an architectural barrier. As the signs in the South once said, "No Colored Served," These barriers say in perhaps a lesser degree of intentional discrimination: "No Disabled Served", "Disabled Need Not Apply", or "Those In Wheelchairs Use Rear Entrance and/or Freight Elevator".

I do not think that anyone really intends to throw water in our faces or to put us down in any way. The problem is that barriers are not even seen by the non-disabled persons, say nothing of wanting to correct them. The tragedy is that they are so easily corrected in the initial design of any building. Mobility independence is the key to making tax payers out of many persons who would otherwise be tax recipients.

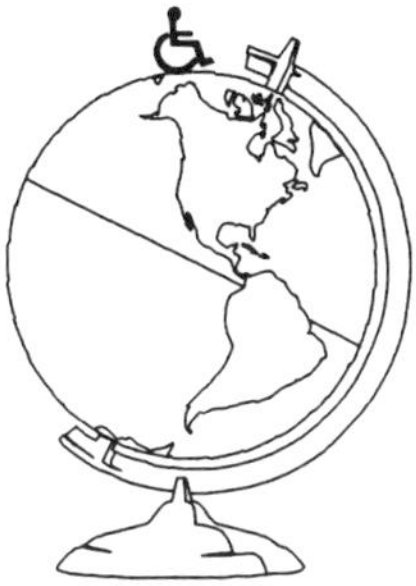

Chapter 4

DISABLED AND THE WORLD

ATTITUDES MAKE THE DIFFERENCE

Let us begin with attitudes toward disability, yours and others. An attitude is your "manner, disposition, feeling, position, etc., toward a person or thing." Most attitude polls use five positions to measure attitude: strongly dislike, dislike, indifferent, like, strongly like, or other terms to indicate feeling or position. Sometimes we have learned our feeling and position from our parents or culture. These are deeply imbedded and die hard. Some we have formed from our own education and experience in life. None of us, including identical twins, has identical parental rearing, culture, education, or experience. Attitudes are uniquely our own, and it is our own attitudes we must confront at this time of adjusting to a disability.

Attitude polls have been conducted on just about every aspect of living, from attitudes on gold in another's teeth (I kid you not) to attitudes relating to the survival of Earth. Sandwiched in between are many polls seeking current attitudes on disability. These attitudes we now want to discuss.

The most common attitudes toward disability that we brought with us into our own disability were feelings of sympathy for, distrust of, and discomfort when faced with another's disability. Those of us who are now disabled, or who are becoming so because of a progressive disorder, are often the captives of our own attitudes regarding disability. A good indicator we have of how we think others feel about us in this new position is to search our memory for how we felt about persons who were disabled before we joined their ranks. Although my personal experience was with a wheelchair, others of you have a similar experience with guide dogs, prostheses, canes, walkers, and the myriad of mobility and life-support mechanisms.

My first time sitting in my wheelchair exposed my own attitude toward disability. It was an exciting day, for my body had been confined to a bed for more than two months since polio. Two therapists lifted my now-skinny torso, while another lifted those useless bird legs and gingerly sat me in my new, shiny wheelchair. They tied me in so I wouldn't fall out and backed away from me so they could see what I looked like sitting up. After a few seconds of jubilation in being free from the bed, the thought crossed my mind: "I don't want anyone to see me in a wheelchair; the hospital staff and patients, and my family are okay, but never a stranger." Five minutes was the limit for the first time up in a wheelchair, and it was back to bed again until tomorrow when perhaps they would allow a few extra minutes.

Why didn't I want anyone to see me in a wheelchair? It was because of an attitude that was carried with me from my first eighteen years to that moment of looking at myself in that wheelchair. Oh, it was okay for other patients to be in wheelchairs; but this was I, Bob, and to me it was at that moment something that negatively set me apart from others outside the protective wall of our hospital. I was overwhelmed by the feeling of shame, having to sit in a wheelchair and not being able to do what the great majority in society could do—walk around without the assistance of any aid or person. A week later that feeling left me, for suddenly I was mobile again and with great effort could at least propel myself slowly down the hallway or around our men's ward. Later it began to dawn on me that there was much more to my disability than just not being able to walk, such as total loss of balance even while sitting.

That negative attitude about wheelchairs, prostheses, canes, oxygen tanks, etc., is common. Is a wheelchair, scooter or any other adaptive device a symbol of giving up? Is it a symbol of mobility? Or is it a symbol of life itself? It is very difficult to dispel the myth of adaptive devices as a sign of giving up. Nowhere has it been so apparent as with those who under some circumstances are somewhat able to function without them, especially disorders such as multiple sclerosis and others that often are progressive. More commonly than not, the family and/or the person with the limitations views a wheelchair or whatever device is used, as a symbol of giving up. Family members often become angry at the users, and the users become angry with themselves.

Passage of time should be able to teach us that these devices are for our comfort, mobility, and for living life to its utmost within the range of our limitations. One time when in my twenties, a well-meaning lady walked over to me in a department store, shook her head with sympathy and said, "Isn't that wheelchair a terrible thing?" For a moment I pondered the question and answered: "No, it is my best friend because I would look awfully silly right now without it." Until we can look at our adaptive devices (those items that set us apart from the great majority in society) as our best friends rather than our enemies, we can only expect others to mirror our negative attitude back to us. The way to change this negativism is first to change our own attitude and watch others respond in like manner.

Do you remember those embarrassing times in life when you did not know how to respond to a person who was blind and you made a terrible slip of the tongue? How about the time the disability was hidden and you made a terrible fax paus? Several times in my life stand out as examples. First on my list is when the person who was blind and who was tuning our family's piano, meticulously removed the keys and set them in order on our dining room table. Being twelve years of age and having an intense curiosity for mechanical devices, I had my nose in the piano as he removed the keys. Suddenly a dime appeared under the now-removed keys. I grabbed it and held it up in front of the piano tuner's face and said, "Look at what I just found." As he stared expressionless, my stomach turned to wax as it came upon me that he could not see the dime. My childhood thoughtlessness had hurt him, I was sure, and I wanted to dive for cover.

Oh, then there was the time a man several blocks away had asked me to service his television. His wife held the door as he pulled me in my wheelchair up the steps into his home. In the dusk I could see this black eye she was sporting and in jest said, "And who hit you in the eye?" Her answer brought that same waxy feeling in my stomach: "No one, it's a birthmark."

Over the years of being in a wheelchair, I have watched others turn white over what was said to me. Most of these have been related to walking or standing of which I can do neither. The most recent was in a counseling session where everything was wrong and nothing could change it. I resorted to comic relief by telling a few Ole and Lena jokes. Both mother and daughter howled with laughter. Then the mother turned serious again and said, "There hasn't been any laughter in this house for many months. You would make a wonderful stand-up comedian." As her voice slowed and trailed off on those last words, her eyes bugged and she thrust her hand over her mouth. I let out with a loud, unceremonious guffaw and we all had another laugh. When talking with those of us who can't walk, stand, see, or hear (or whatever we can't do), these become frightening words to those who can.

Now for those who have a choice of when to use a wheelchair or other device, know that there are times when you should and times when you should not use your device. A wheelchair or scooter in particular can be a seemingly legitimate excuse for the lazy or undriven, and in some cases it truly is a symbol of giving up. In that situation the device is bad for us because giving up is bad. The day we give up is the day we begin to deteriorate. One day an auto-parts counter man carried some heavy parts to my car for me. As I struggled to get in he asked if he could help me, but I politely refused his assistance. He became very angry and snorted, "You never let anyone help you." My response was simply this: "Bernie, the day that I allow someone to do for me what I can and should do for myself is the day that I begin to die." He looked surprised, thought for a moment and muttered, "I see what you mean."

The other side of the coin reflects the decision of some of us to not use our devices when we should use them. Persons with multiple sclerosis are particularly vulnerable to this mistake. Many can walk short distances but are unsteady on their feet. In their attempt to not give up and/or to look normal in a crowd, they choose to walk. So often this leads to disaster because you will learn that the crowd does not notice that you must hang on to a wall or someone's arm. They do not see the cane or the halting gait. They look straight ahead and push off to their destination. Unfortunately, they sometimes bump or brush you over, and there you are, a pile on the floor. There is shame on your part, horror on theirs, and what could have been a pleasing experience for all those affected turns into a nightmare.

Do yourself a favor when going shopping or knowingly into any type of crowd—use your wheelchair or scooter. If the distances you must walk cause your legs to weaken or give you shortness of breath—use your own, a rented, or a borrowed wheelchair. Is this clear? It is very selfish for us to create a hazard or to make those in our group wait for us to rest simply because of our pride. Wisely use a wheelchair!

Let me warn you that you are not even safe encased in fifty pounds of steel and wheels. Now you would think that a wheelchair, of all things, would be obvious to anyone in a crowd. However, when folk have their minds and their eyes set on something other than the surprise obstacle of a person encased in steel sitting quietly on the sidelines or moving down an aisle, anything can happen and it usually does.

I have had some bone crushing and also some delightful ladies trip on my footrests and end up in my lap. Also there have been many times that I have apologized for my footrests sticking out and tripping some poor soul who only saw the top of my head and didn't pay any attention to the whereabouts of the rest of me. Although they should have been more alert, nonetheless, I felt badly that my chair had caused them a possible physical or emotional jar. Generally, society is not intentionally thoughtless, so it does become our problem to be thoughtful and careful of others so that we are not bumped or dumped. It is unfortunate for all when we have the attitude, "Well, here I am, I have a perfect right to be here, and it is their problem if they don't recognize the hazard of my device."

Up to this point we have talked more about attitudes toward wheelchairs, etc., but it is important to realize that our attitude toward any of these devices is a reflection of our attitudes on disability as a whole. The general attitude of society toward persons with disabilities is much more positive than most of us suspect. If the general population is characteristic of college students responding to one study, society expects us to be above average in being conscientious, self-reliant, kind, persistent, alert, creative, religious, impulsive, and unselfish. We were rated average in being friendly, trustworthy, emotionally stable, tolerant, courageous, and submissive; having self-pity, social poise, vitality, and self-confidence. Aha, but we were rated below average in emotional release, realism/reverie, aggressiveness, social adaptability (difficult adjusting to new situations), and sensitiveness.

Then there is our own attitude toward ourselves and our disability. Rather than quoting so-called studies, the following attitudes are gleaned from my own experience with myself and thousands of those with whom I have counseled. Remember, we are all individuals and there will be exceptions, but as a general rule persons with disabilities look on themselves and their limitations a bit differently than does society.

We tend to think of ourselves much more negatively than we did before we were disabled, or in the case of one with a congenital disability (one at birth or early in childhood), more negatively than we would have had we not been disabled. A disability truly is ego threatening. In all my years as a counselor of persons with disabilities, the most common problem we face is low self-esteem or low self-image. Surprisingly, this is the same problem faced by the general population, so we are not alone in our low opinion of self.

If the general population suffers from low self image, would you not expect those with a disability to have an even lower opinion of themselves than if they were able bodied or able minded? Unfortunately, one's relative position in society seems to be established by what we can do, how much money we earn, and how much we can accumulate from what we earn. That leaves most of us who have disabilities in the dust, doesn't it?

Well, yes and no. The answer is no if you learn to make comparisons of yourself with yourself and not someone else. If we have a physical disability and compare ourselves with our able-bodied co-workers in any type of physical task, we will naturally come up short—and down goes our self esteem. If we are intellectually limited and compare ourselves to our neighbor, Mr. Average, we will grit our teeth in disgust over our lack of performance. Give us intellectually-disabled persons a physical task and we just might shine. Give us physically disabled persons an intellectual task and we just might shine. We may just even do better than our able-bodied/able-minded co-workers or neighbor, but does that make us better than they? You say, "Of course not, for we all have strengths and weaknesses."

Do you realize what you just said? "He or she is not less of a person because I can beat that person at Trivial Pursuit, Scrabble, or whatever." Now turn that around: "I am not less of a person because someone can outperform me in any or all areas. I am not less of a person because of color, race, disability, social or cultural background, or anything else. My worth is related to my ability to be kind, helpful, thoughtful, and to give love and receive it." That same yardstick should have been used to evaluate our worth before we became disabled, and it should be used by every person on the face of this earth.

If you are an able-bodied yuk, you are a yuk; if you are a disabled yuk, you are a yuk. Make no mistake that in either case you are a yuk. If you are an able-bodied kind, thoughtful, considerate, generous, helpful, loving person; you have a great deal of worth. If you are a kind, thoughtful, considerate, generous, helpful, loving person who happens to be disabled, you have as much worth as the so-called able-bodied or able-minded person with these same characteristics. Personal worth is not what we can do, but it is what we are—and don't you ever forget that. The most severe disability need not prevent us from being truly worthwhile persons, and we should strive to improve our worth.

The negative traits that I see cropping up in those of us with disabilities may be characteristic of persons with disabilities, but they need not be so. These are being selfish and self-centered, manipulating others by using our disability, lacking assertiveness and aggressiveness, wallowing in self-pity, entertaining unrealistic goals, and expecting the world to bow at our feet and serve us because we have been inconvenienced by a disability. These attitudes hurt us in all relationships with family, friends, and society. For our own good we must keep these in mind and do what we can to change them.

Let's conclude this attitude section by going back and picking up one word we used early in this section. That word is SHAME. Sure, I was ashamed for a week thinking of outsiders seeing me in a wheelchair, but that should be a very passing feeling. I could not help my condition, and you cannot help yours either. As long as we do the best we can with what we have, we should feel no shame. Anything less than our best, as with any non-disabled person, should be and is shameful.

The most hurtful of all shame is when our spouse, our family, our friends, or someone whom we love or care about has the unfortunate feeling of shame for us simply because we have a disability. There are husbands who will not go out to dinner or any other place to be seen in public with their wives of whom they are ashamed simply on the basis of a disability. There are wives, children, and others who feel ashamed of us (or is it for us) when we are in the public eye. If there is any shame for anything it should be if we behave in a shameful manner—angry, rude, arrogant, distasteful, or any socially-unacceptable behavior.

Some disabilities make eating or drinking gracefully very difficult. If that be our lot, let us be considerate of how we may affect others and locate ourselves in an area which provides the most privacy. Some persons are not able to tolerate poor table etiquette even when they understand it is a result of our disability. However, it should be our goal to improve any part of our behavior that will lend to a greater social acceptance, whether it be a simple smile or a wiped chin.

We also have the responsibility to learn how those close to us feel about our disability and how to handle the new situations that will come up in our lives. The first step is to let them know exactly how we feel about our disability. They have no way of knowing how they should look at us until they know how we look at ourselves. Be honest and straightforward. This should put them at rest and you can begin to openly discuss the new rules of your relationship. Ask and expect to be treated like anyone else.

Keep in mind you are just one spoke in the family wheel and not the hub. Everything the family does should not revolve around you and your limitations. Should your husband give up his favorite sport because you no longer can be a part of it? Should your wife spend every waking hour taking care of your needs? If you want to see a family or friendship disintegrate, just make sure that it revolves around you and your disability. Talk about it and keep reminding them what you cannot do. Make them feel guilty for not wanting to cater to your every whim. Are some disabled persons like that?

Absolutely, and there is a continual string of them seeking my counsel and asking why their relationships are falling apart.

A major goal for you is to try to understand other's reactions to your condition. Perhaps this is the first time one has seen you since your accident or illness. They may be unable to cover their shock or their deep emotional feelings. My first Thanksgiving after polio found me with our family at my aunt's and uncle's home. The men had to carry me up seven steps and then out again down seven steps. In the confusion of leaving, my mother forgot her purse in the house and had to retrieve it after I was loaded into the car. When she went back into the house, there was a living room full of relatives all crying. They had held back their emotions until they thought we were safely out of sight. Until you have been in a similar situation and hurt so badly for someone you loved, you cannot understand the hurt (sometimes uncontrollable) others feel for you.

Now all the responsibility for understanding does not fall on your shoulders; it also rests with the family and close friends, and in a sense on society as well. You and your intimate circle of family and friends must learn together that in the new situation, much of what you once did is no longer possible. As mentioned in another chapter, John Ritter played in a great movie titled "Leave Yesterday Behind." This movie was the story of a man who became a paraplegic in a horse accident, and before he could successfully face the world again he had to give up yesterday's ideals and dreams.

I gave up dreams; you must give up dreams and look at today and tomorrow rather than yesterday. It is not easy, and some never achieve this; neither do they achieve contentedness in their lives. We are playing a new game of life, and we had better realize that with a new game comes new rules. You must acquaint yourself with these rules. There will be many changes in your life, but in the end you can win and be successful in living life to its fullest within your limitations.

ATTITUDE—by Charles Swindoll

> "The longer I live, the more I realized the impact of attitude on life. Attitude, to me, is more important than the past, than education, than money, than circumstances, than failures, than successes, than what other people think or say or

do. It is more important than appearance, giftedness, or skill. It will make or break a company—a church—a home. The remarkable thing is we have a choice every day regarding the attitude we will embrace for that day. We cannot change our past—we cannot change the fact that people will act in a certain way. We cannot change the inevitable. The only thing we can do is play on the one string we have, and that is our attitude. I am convinced that life is 10% what happens to me and 90% how I react to it. And so it is with you. We are in charge of our Attitudes."

Celebrating A Disability

Have you ever thought about celebrating your disability? In my pre-polio days in Minnesota, October and November were exciting months. October offered the opportunity for duck and pheasant hunting. Waiting for the legal opening of any particular hunting season, it was so exciting that my arms and my gun would shake uncontrollably. November usually brought the first cold that would freeze our pond for skating. Often the early ice was so thin that it would have broken if I hadn't kept moving, and sometimes the ice that I had skated upon early in the morning was gone by the time I came home from high school.

To me, August and September were the least exciting months of the year. In fact, they were downright unpleasant. This was the time of the year that allergies—asthma and hay fever—brought me to a miserable and sudden stop. While the other kids were playing football I was trapped indoors wheezing. While the other kids were excitedly running up and down the stairs on the first days of school, I was taking time out on the landings to use my inhaler to make it to the top.

As a young person the "dog days" of August contained very little happiness for me, and it was fitting that it was in August that polio changed all the months of the year for the remainder of my life. If our disability came upon us as an adolescent or adult, that month of loss often becomes a memorial to what we were. August of 1993 was celebrated as my 47th anniversary of not standing up.

Do I mean celebrated as some sort of sarcasm or cynicism for what polio took from me? No, I truly celebrate. On my 25th anniversary of "not walking," my wife and I went out to dinner. The waitress somehow overheard my comments to Janice about this being a celebration and risked the question, "Is this your anniversary," to which I nodded my head and said, "Yup, 25 years." She smiled sweetly and said that it was her privilege to serve us on our 25th wedding anniversary. You should have seen the look on her face when I corrected her and said, "No, this is not our wedding anniversary but rather that of 25 years of sitting on my butt." She didn't know where to look or what to say. Is that shock what one would expect from a celebration of disability?

Well, first of all it was a celebration of living. At that time I had lived 25 years longer than had been expected in those early weeks of polio when the lives of many of us hung in the balances. It was a celebration of a great marriage, two children, and a life-long ministry specializing in counsel to persons with disabilities as well as their families. Had there been a choice would I have opted for not being disabled? You bet I would, but there were no options. However, you can see that there were some compensations that helped even the score.

Another of the compensations of my disability was that it helped me get my priorities in order—what is really important in life. Is it having money and material things? Is it having a prestigious job, position, or place to live? Is it having the right automobile or knowing the right people? For me it became none of that. Rather it has just been a peaceful contentment with what and who I am.

No matter what type and degree of disability we have, there are none of us who cannot contribute something to another's life. Little do we know what these contributions have been or what they will be. It may just be a smile at a stranger. You may have turned a life completely around and not known it. It just may be that because of you someone got a new arrangement of priorities that changed his or her life. Contentment comes from the inside out, not from the outside in. It is not related to the condition of our bodies. In my case it came from a commitment to Jesus Christ and a commitment to Christian service. My contentment is in knowing that in some small way my life has been useful to someone other than myself.

WELL, WHAT ELSE CAN WE DO?

Actually, the list would be shorter of what we cannot do. If you name some seemingly-impossible task for someone with your limitations, we can most likely find someone with similar limitations who has accomplished this feat. Of course there are things that we cannot do, and in my case it would be anything that absolutely required the use of legs and/or balance. What we don't realize is that many times there are ways—creative ways—of doing the same thing in a different way. It is on the order of putting five nickels in the pay phone rather than one quarter. Creative minds have the edge in accomplishing the seemingly impossible.

Some of us may want to do what appears to be extremely difficult or even impossible to make us appear to be less disabled than others think we are. Some of us want to prove to ourselves that our disability is conquered. Some feel that by doing normal things we somehow will be viewed as more normal. Some simply need the experience to enhance their egos. However, some accomplish these tasks simply because if we are to live life we must do them.

First of all, let me tell you that it has never been my desire to be noted for physical or mental feats accomplished in spite of my limitations. I do not see them as anything unusual, just an out-of-the-ordinary approach to solving problems. However, those close to me felt that some of these solutions might be encouraging to those of you who may want to become creative with your new environment. These are only being used as examples of what can be done in spite of a severe disability (medical evaluation, not mine). It is not implied that if I could do it, you could also. It must be remembered that you may be able to do some things that I cannot even though we may have similar limitations. The key to accomplishment is drive and skill. It is my goal to challenge both your drive and your skill to sometimes solve the unsolvable.

Somehow some of my unusual solutions have been picked up by the news media in its search for human interest stories and have often appeared in their columns along with a picture to two. "That guy in a wheelchair who lives across the street must be nuts." I am sure that has been said over some of my crazy stunts. What is about to be told is not necessarily sensible, but it was something I had to do.

My very first hurdle was learning how to get into the car without assistance and being able to pull my wheelchair in after me. In those early days (and to some extent today) the rehabilitation thrust was to teach us how to walk, even though it was evident that for many of us it was impossible. There was no thought about teaching us the "Activities of Daily Living." What we learned of those ADL we each learned on our own. Perhaps that encouraged many of us to challenge our new environment.

At the time I learned to get myself and my wheelchair in and out of an automobile without assistance, it was considered an impossibility with my limitations. These were the days before electric or hydraulic wheelchair lifts. On my first attempt I slid out of my chair onto the car floor and then pulled, pushed, twisted, turned, and grunted my way up into the seat. If I was going to drive and be independent, this was a must. At that time there were no commercial hand controls available. There was no automatic transmission on this car so I had to perform all driving tasks with my two hands that normally had been done with two hands and two feet. My first custom hand controls utilized two vacuum valves to activate the clutch and brakes, and a lever for the throttle. What a mechanical monstrosity, but to the amazement of many, my independence was guaranteed.

Steps were always a challenge. Most persons are surprised to learn that there are no functional chair-climbing wheelchairs. They are usually a giant imitation of a child's wind-up army tank with rubber tracks. One of those first feats to getting down steps was to learn to balance on the large rear wheels (pop a wheelie), move slowly up to the curb, and then drop with a thump down into the street. If the step treads (the part on which you plant your feet) were at least 14" deep, it was possible, using the precision of a high-wire performer, to drop down any number of them. However, if balance was lost it would have been a catastrophe, and I chose not to take that risk.

There were many times in my post-polio life in which stairs presented the ultimate problem. Many of us paraplegics learned to "fanny" stairs by lifting or lowering ourselves one at a time, and then getting back in our chairs at the top or bottom of the stairs. However, most of us needed someone to take the wheelchair up or down for us. Some leg amputees become very adept at both fannying and pulling the chair up. Once in a pinch, I tied a rope around my waist and to the chair at the bottom, then fannied the steps to the top and pulled my chair up after me.

More than once in a mall or store I was scolded by security personnel for risking my life and their jobs by taking the escalator either up or down. Up was easier because all I had to do was position myself before the rising steps and wheel on at the right moment, then grab the moving handrails and literally hang on for dear life. Going down was more precarious in that I had to do the proverbial "wheelie" and move out onto the descending step at *precisely* the right micro-second, having only about one inch of tolerance between success and disaster. Then it was necessary to balance carefully on two wheels all the way to the bottom where I usually met up with scowling, scolding security people. My answer usually was, "Please show me the state statute that prohibits me from using the escalator." In my old age it is yet commonplace for me to take the UP-escalator, but the challenge of the down one has been passed off to those younger of heart and quicker reaction time. My wife added this line: "Please don't try this—it is a stupid, inconsiderate thing to do." Well, that puts me in my place, but I must concede that she is correct.

Steps again were my greatest challenge, not climbing them but building them. We had a two story house in which I did much of the interior. How does a paralyzed man build steps? First of all the stair stringers (the sawtooth 2x12s you nail the steps to) had to be cut and nailed into place. Then the stair treads cut and nailed. Although being around carpenters all my life I had never figured and cut my own stringers. That was a mathematical nightmare, but they were designed, cut, and nailed in place.

Then it was measuring and cutting a stair tread (the piece that you step on) and the riser (the vertical piece your toe hits) and nailing them in place. That was for two steps until I no longer could reach. So it was out of my chair onto the step that had just been installed and lift myself into position to measure, fanny down the new stairs, cut, and fanny back up to nail and measure. This went on until I was at the top. This was the greatest challenge of my life and there was no one around to see me do it or help me. If you are familiar with carpentry, you should ask one question, and that is how I managed to secure those stringers at the top of the stairs four feet above my reach before I began the tread/riser cutting and nailing process. That is another story.

Six years earlier this problem of reaching the ceiling had been solved so that I could nail and tape wallboard as well as do the house wiring. Out of 2x4s and a hydraulic bumper jack came my first "high chair." I lifted my butt to the arm of my wheelchair and then transferred onto a seat about three feet off the ground that was able to be jacked up so that the ceiling was in reach. It looked much like an oversized electric chair used for capital punishment, but it was on casters and rolled me around where I needed to go. My wife and I sheet-rocked, taped, and wired the entire house.

The newspaper got a hold of that one and it was teletyped around the country. Most who read it did not believe it, but that was okay with me. When being introduced to a group of disabled Vietnam War veterans, the social worker began her introduction by saying, "On the bulletin board you most likely have seen the story of the man in a wheelchair who constructed most of his own house...." However before she could introduce me as that man, the vets said almost in unison, "That's a bunch of bull s---."

For reasons of economy, we had a second floor in our new home and a stairway to get there. Of course that was no help to me, so in the design which I had drawn there was an opening for an elevator shaft. Makes sense, but not when the price of a commercial elevator and installation was known.

Back to the drawing board to design a low-cost elevator. The elevator car was cut and welded (having learned those skills along life's road), rails were drilled and positioned in the shaft to guide the car. I made a series of sheaves and used a cable and gear-reduction motor. My wife hauled the cable and pulleys to the attic, secured them and dropped the cable. After this mechanism was attached to the motor and the elevator car, the next step was to secure those car rails that were above my reach. This was possible by getting my wheelchair on the car and running it up the rails, one foot at a time, securing them with large screws as I went.

In 1973 we moved to Phoenix and my trusty old 2x4 "highchair" was too heavy and awkward to move. A new one was constructed out of steel, this time designed so that my wheelchair could be backed onto the platform and a battery-powered winch would move me up and down. It had easy-roll casters like the old one, but this one would take me at least a foot higher and I didn't need to struggle to get on and off. To this day it serves me well. It has allowed me to remodel the entire interior of our home here in Phoenix as well as lay hundreds of concrete blocks that were higher than I could normally reach from my wheelchair.

Nutty? Perhaps, but it was my way of getting the most out of life. Most of these things I have done have not necessarily been sensible, but I fortunately had the challenge, the skills, and an almost-foolish drive for independence. Your challenge and your skills will be different from mine.

There are artists such as Joni Eareckson Tada who are quadriplegics and who paint with brushes in their mouths—not just passable art, but prize-winning art competitive in the world of art. It is not just excellent because it is painstakingly done with a brush in one's mouth; it is excellent because it is excellent art—period.

Some paraplegics choose to compete in all sorts of athletic events. Some climb mountains; some race in marathons. The media consistently makes us aware of those persons who with some severe limitations have performed the impossible. If the world of the able-bodied does it, we will do it, perhaps differently and perhaps more labored and more slowly—but one or more of us will do it.

Don't sell yourself short, for if you do you will find yourself short—short of life's satisfactions. However, don't ever be tricked into believing the great American lie, that if you want anything badly enough and try hard enough you will succeed. That is true only if that something is within the true possibilities of our limitations. However, until we attempt something we have no idea if it is out of reach.

Doctors, Hospitals, and Medical Practitioners

When this was suggested as a topic for this book, it was my inner feeling to ignore it. Medical personnel are often so encumbered by the medical aspect of disability, they have little time or feeling for the emotional aspect. Ask any medical doctor if the mind plays an important role in the healing and rehabilitation process and he will answer with an emphatic, yes. The doctor is well aware of the body/mind relationship, but so often there is little time spent learning about and dealing with the emotions. If a disabled person exhibits serious symptoms of maladjustment, he is referred to a psychiatrist. My experience has been that few psychiatrists have an accurate appraisal of the effects a disability has on the emotions. Therefore, they will tend to use analysis and treatment that may work on the general population, but not in the specialized area of disability.

To really appreciate the emotional stress a disability places on us, one must have been there himself or have had many years of experience specializing in disability. There will be arguments on this, but it is simply my observation as well as of many persons with disabilities who have sought the help of mental-health professionals.

It is a common myth among the medical personnel that a disability automatically distorts our view of life and there can never be perfect adjustment, only an improvement. We are expected to think and behave in certain ways, and when we appear to be normal in our emotions and behavior, the psychological world seems surprised. Many times my professional mental-health co-workers have been amazed to the point of mentioning to me how surprised they are at how normal and well-adjusted I am (whatever that means).

So often at city, state, and national meetings relating to rehabilitation, disabled clergypersons are sought to bring the invocation. Back a number of years ago the program chairperson of the Governor's Commission on the Employment of the Handicapped in the State of Minnesota was discussing this plight with me. Suddenly her mouth fell open and she stammered, "Why is it that I never thought of you? I just never think of you as handicapped." Perhaps I acted too normal and well adjusted to be disabled, but regardless, I accepted it as a compliment.

No, disability need not relegate us to the behavioral scrap heap. If those of you in the medical world can understand that we are grieving for a loss of a body and its functions as seriously as one can grieve for a loss of a spouse, it can help you better understand our behavior. Somewhere out there is the reality of what we can do—spare us the myths of automatic behavioral maladjustment and that we should have every possible treatment available.

Persons who are blind shouldn't expect sighted people to understand the world of the blind; and persons paralyzed by disabilities shouldn't expect "walking" people to understand the world of the non-walking. What we do expect is to be asked for advice on how it is best to handle our unmanageable bodies when being placed on an X-ray table or examining table. Isn't it sad that I know of only one local medical doctor who has an examining table that can be lowered to wheelchair height and raised to the doctor's height by the touch of a button. Doctors, they are available.

And how about doctors offices? There are doors that are too narrow or awkward for wheelchairs to enter the examining room or the toilet. At one of my doctor's offices there are no steps, but a ramp more than two times the acceptable standard of one foot rise in twelve feet, and I have all I can do to get up the thing. In the doctor's offices as well as the world at large, the equipment is designed for able-bodied, agile, standing, mobile persons.

Technology has made many things more possible today in the world of reconstructive surgery and other areas of rehabilitation. However, one thing that continues to be lacking seems to me to be reality. You continue to spend time and precious dollars attempting to do what you know (or should know) is impossible. Perhaps it is your inexperience or it is because your profession cannot tolerate the thought that there comes a time when nothing further can be done. Perhaps by continuing treatment that is not effective or that has become ineffective, you have a sense of release from responsibility because you are doing everything possible.

Please be careful how you encourage or discourage us. What you tell us, especially in those early months, is accepted as "gospel" truth. One of our problems is that we believe you because this is all so new to us. Most likely we will accept your attitude toward our disability just as others will accept our attitude toward our own disability. We are tender people and to have you walk into our hospital room and say, "Well, you might as well face the fact that you are never going to walk again," as a friend of mine was told, borders on cruelty.

Another personal friend of mine was told by a physical therapist that she would only live perhaps twelve to fifteen years after polio. She accepted this "professional" appraisal of her life span and went home hoping she would live long enough to rear her three young children. All of her planning for life was colored by this myth. She is yet alive and well forty-plus years later being concerned with each of her six grandchildren.

You may argue that this took place back in 1950 and it would not happen today. Well, how about another example from 1980. I received a call from a woman with multiple sclerosis who was told that she had been given five years to live. These five years had now passed and she was frantic at the prospects of dying and leaving her husband and a six year old child. What cruelty! She did not die then or ten years later. However, she suffered all the pangs of death because of a foolish statement.

If you don't have the time or the ability to deliver the so-called message of doom diplomatically, find someone who is capable of doing it. Perhaps we need more hospital chaplains trained in this area. Discuss it with the family because in most cases there is more hurt that needs attention in the waiting room than on the surgery table. We have specially-trained persons for everything else in our rehabilitation process, how about beginning the procedure with a qualified clergyman, social worker or someone who understands *and* cares. Is that asking too much?

Always leave room for a thread of realistic hope, as mentioned earlier, the *Bible* reads, *"Without a vision* (hope), *the people perish."* Be honest within reason, but give us our odds, be it one-in-ten or one-in-a-billion. Given time, our bodies and our minds will heal to their capacities. Given time, our minds and hearts will adjust the odds to our own reality.

Chapter 5

Limits to Independence

ARCHITECTURAL BARRIERS

Just what do we mean by an architectural barrier? It is simply any obstacle in a man-designed facility that prevents or hinders the accessibility of any person to use the building or facility for that which it was designed. This includes anything in the construction of a building (residential or commercial) including its entrance/exit to the area to or from which a person with a disability must travel when using either public or private transportation.

Should someone who has no mobility limitations be concerned with architectural barriers? Absolutely! Should you be so fortunate as to have no limitation now, that does not mean you will not be limited tomorrow. No one in our family had any mobility limitation until I contracted polio. The family home was a nightmare. It had a street-level driveway with a walk-out basement/garage. This required everyone to walk the curved, steeply-inclined sidewalk to the back porch that boasted five steps. It was also a two story home with three bedrooms upstairs. The bathroom was totally inaccessible for a wheelchair. The professionals were called in but had no solutions, not even the possibility of an outside elevator. The only solution was a new home without these barriers, and it was a costly move. In my years of counseling I have seen this same scene repeated many times over—a new disability in an incompatible home.

Keep in mind that what is good for me and other persons with these limitations in mobility is good for those of you who are not at this moment so encumbered. If you live long enough you will be limited. Those curb cuts, handicapped parking spaces, ramps, wider doors, grab bars, etc., will in the end greatly enhance the quality of your life. All of us should think l-o-n-g r-a-n-g-e. End up in a wheelchair or on crutches for any reason even for a few weeks and you will learn the value of preventing or removing these barriers *before* they are barriers.

This list does not include commercial barriers such as drinking fountains that are too high, phone booths that are inaccessible, rest room impossibilities, aisles too narrow, doors too difficult to open. Would you not think that hospitals would be barrier free? Strangely, they are often among the worst offenders. One new hospital I visited had a nice, concrete ramp up to the front of the building. There was a substantial railing on the side of the ramp and the entrance doors were wide and easy to open. However (can you believe this?), just inside those easy-to-open doors were three unramped steps.

Here are some of the more common household architectural barriers:

1. Steps of any height. That means no sunken living rooms.
2. Thresholds or other extremely sharp inclines of one-half inch or more. Front casters on most wheelchairs cannot climb these without excessive effort.
3. Narrow doorways: entrance doors, interior doors (especially bathroom doors). No doorway should be less than 36 inches. A 30-inch doorway will allow the average adult wheelchair of 26 inches to pass, but it is a knuckle buster. Forgotten is the fact that a 30-inch door does not give a 30-inch opening, but rather about 27 inches.
4. Narrow hallways: The wheelchair standard is for wall-to-wall width to be 4 feet or wider. Why should that be when most wheelchairs are only about 26 inches wide? It is because you cannot negotiate a sharp turn into a bedroom without skinning knuckles and knocking off pieces of the door, its casing and jamb. In many cases these turns cannot be negotiated unless someone gets behind your wheelchair and lifts the back end and slides it into a position directly facing the opening.
5. Any sharp turns in hallways or on ramps. Would it surprise you to learn that it takes an empty 5′ by 5′ of floor space (25 square feet) to turn a standard wheelchair around without difficulty.

6. Any fixed cabinet in a kitchen or bathroom that prevents a wheelchair user from wheeling directly up to the sink, range, washbowl, or toilet.
7. Fixed faucets on kitchen sink, bathroom lavatory, tub or shower, or flush lever or button on a toilet that is difficult to operate for persons who have limited use of hands, arms, or shoulders.
8. A lipped entrance to shower stall preventing shower chair from moving easily into the stall.
9. Bathtubs and showers without safety or lift grab bars.
10. Plush and/or thickly-padded carpets.

You most likely have seen from this list that there are many barriers in the home or office that restrict or hamper movement of persons with disabilities that are not commonly thought to be such. If one can bump, grind or wiggle the person into a room, it is okay. Wrong! It is degrading and demoralizing to have someone assist us in doing what we should be able to do for ourselves had these restrictions or barriers been removed.

It takes time and effort on the part of the care giver or physical assistant that should be utilized on other things that the person with the disability cannot do. In other words, you have wasted a valuable resource of time and energy simply because these barriers prevented the person with the disability from doing them by him or herself. When we must ask for help in doing any task it is a reminder of our disability. Please do everything in your power to provide a barrier-free environment for your loved one.

Possible Solutions And Alternatives

Well, what can you do? Most of us who became disabled lived in a home in which most or all of the above architectural barriers were present. We come home from the nightmare of facing our disability to a nightmare of facing a hostile environment in our once-friendly home. When designing and building a new home most of these barriers can be remedied at a very small cost.

For example, in a new home the grading can be raised at entrance doors to eliminate or make shorter ramps and/or with less incline. All doors can be prescribed to be 36 inches (or 3′0″ in trade language). Hallways can be wide with no sharp turns. Bathrooms can have backing for grab bars placed between the studs when roughing in or framing the house. The ideal is to start from scratch, but often circumstances make this impossible.

However, in many cases these modifications to remove barriers already in place are costly. For example, if you are building a house, a 36-inch door and frame will be in the neighborhood of $15-$20 over the cost of one 30 inches wide. Making this change later can easily run $300-$500 for a single opening. Everything done after the house is built will be many times greater than if it had been included in the design and building.

Pre-1980 homes often use standard framing construction in which the interior walls bear part of the roof weight. If the home uses the now-common roof trusses, the cost of widening a door opening is less because the wall on either side of the door header does not require building-code changes that are required for any modification of a load-bearing wall. There are some cheaper solutions such as special offset hinges for doors. These hinges move the hinge-side of the door out of the opening and give a potential extra 1-3/8 inches in width.

Ramps are the easiest and cheapest items to construct. If possible they should have no turns and should have a rise or incline of not more that 1 foot in 12 feet. For a 2-foot rise the ramp should be 24 feet long, and if for a 3-foot rise it should be 36 feet long. A single 4-inch step requires a ramp 4 feet long. Don't kid yourself into thinking this is not necessary or that you can skimp. Without further discussion, just believe me.

Another forgotten item in ramps is to include a level platform long enough for the wheelchair to sit while the user puts key in door and opens it. No platform—whee, the wheelchair and user can take a quick and dangerous ride to the bottom. If the entrance door opens into the building, the ramp platform needs only to be 3 feet in length. If the door opens outward or has a storm door that opens outward, the platform must be 6 feet in length.

In newer homes it has become the custom to install high thresholds so that the doors will clear any thick carpet or pad installed. The object is to not have to send a carpenter back to have doors cut off. That's fine if you can lift your feet. Thresholds can be purchased at any hardware or builders' supply that range from 5/8" to 1-3/4" high. However if you install a lower threshold, what are you going to do with the gaping opening under the door that was previously covered by the high threshold? You must either buy a new door and have it hung, or you must take off the old one and add material to the bottom of the door. Neither is cheap, but it is better than a constant struggle for the remainder of your life in that house.

BATHROOMS

The placement of the toilet in the bathroom is very important. However, unless you want to remodel the entire bathroom that would include the tub/shower and lavatory/cabinets, don't even think of moving the toidy bowl. It is better to leave all fixtures where they are and design cabinets around them, change the location of the door opening, or even move a wall that does not include plumbing. Grab bars are also important around the toilet, bathtub and shower. As with all grab-bar installations, they must be anchored to "the Rock of Gibraltar."

Unless you require a custom-shaped bar, it can be purchased much more cheaply in places like K-Mart. They come in even-foot sizes for much less than half the price of custom bars. I paid $90 for one for our bathtub that was in the shape of an L for going around the back of the tub. Two single bars, 3′ and 2′ from K-Mart would have done the same trick for less than $25. Also keep in mind the diameter of the bar is important. The smaller the diameter of the bar, the better the grip for fingers, but also strength is greatly sacrificed. Use smaller diameter bars for pulling on and larger ones for lifting from.

Neither plaster nor plaster board (sheetrock) has any strength of its own and cannot bear weight. Make sure you are in a stud and use #12 screws (or larger) that are at least 1-3/4" long. If no stud exists where it is needed, it is possible to install a 2x4 on the wall to the studs and then anchor the grab bars to the 2x4 as illustrated on the following page. When installing the 2x4, use 1/4" or 5/16" lag screws (with flat washers) that are no less that 3-1/2" long but preferably 4" long. Know that the installation of grab or lift bars to 2x4s won't enhance the beauty of your bathroom. However, it is functional and it is safe, for it is much wiser to not sacrifice safety for beauty. If beauty is really important to you, cut up the wall and get some heavy backing material behind it for the supports. In place of a 2x4, you may substitute a piece of flat steel ¼" thick by whatever width necessary (most likely 3" to 4" wide). Use #12x2" to secure steel to studs, using two screws on each stud rather than the one lag screw prescribed for the 2x4. The grab-bar flange must be secured to the steel by drilling holes and tapping them with the proper threads. The steel can be painted your bathroom colors.

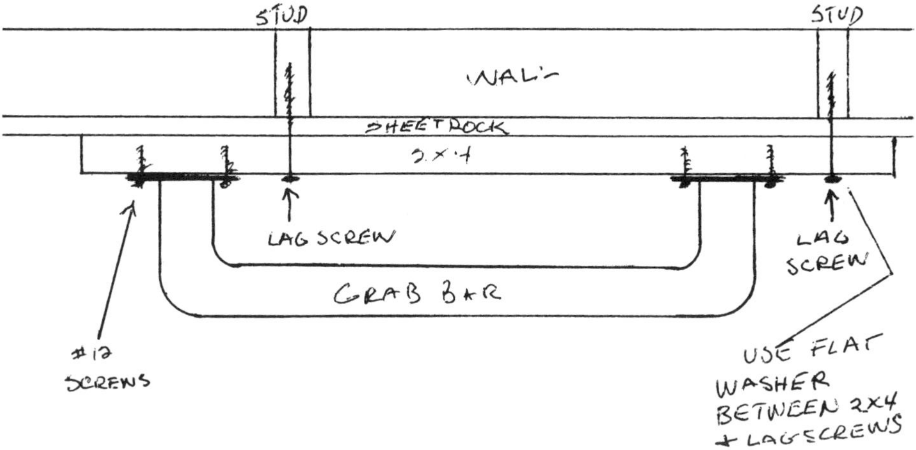

You might think that if you are lifting or pulling on a grab bar, it needs a more secure anchor into the wall than it would if you just use it to give steadiness as you get in and out, up or down, or on and off. However, if you should lose your balance or footing, it may be required to hold all your weight. Any grab bar that you use would of necessity need to support 100% of your weight. Grab bars can work loose from use and will be very dangerous. Do not use a grab bar that has even the slightest movement. It must be firm!

A grab bar is a grab bar? It must be remembered that a grab bar and its installation are as unique as dentures are to its wearer. One size does not fit all; in fact, dentures cannot be exchanged between people. Although your grab bars may give me some assistance, they may also be a total detriment. The two areas of greatest need are the bathtub/shower and the misnamed piece of pottery called the toilet (the correct name for a toilet is *water closet*, a wash bowl is a *lavatory*.)

When installing a grab bar use your physics sense (not related to actual *bowel* activities) for the best and needed leverage. If possible have someone make a cheap model out of 2x4s or pipe that can be safely used but also modified easily until the best placement is discerned. Keep in mind that muscles have their greatest strength in certain positions. If bars are placed on either or both sides of the water closet for assisting one to lift themselves to a standing position, it depends upon which part of the operation needs the most leverage advantage that determines optimum placement. It is really a cut-and-try situation. Poorly-positioned bars are sometimes worse than none at all.

There are some adjustable bars for around the toilet. (Ah, shucks, I might as well give in and call it the toilet—everyone else does but plumbers.) They are welded to straps that rest directly on the floor. The bars can be adjusted for height and there is no drilling on the walls. However, some locations for these bars can make it quite inconvenient for some of the able-bodied persons. Keep in mind there is no perfect solution in which everyone is happy. The priority should be to make a happy person out of the one who would otherwise need assistance, or who is playing loosely with safety.

The great and wonderful government bureaucracies and the barrier committees tried to set up standards for all of the barriers we have mentioned. Unfortunately, they tried to be all things to all people. Have you ever tried to sit on one of those toilets in commercial or interstate highway rest rooms? Whoever came up with that height ought to have his head examined. Sure it might benefit 5% of the disabled population but hinders 95%. Dare I say it? When it comes time for the paper work, one usually leans over left, right, or forward to make way for the operation. If one is paralyzed, perched on a *throne* on which your feet can't reach the floor, you are in precarious trouble. Not only that, if you sit more than a few minutes your circulation is cut off in your legs and they go to sleep. What you don't need in extracting yourself from a toilet is sleeping legs. Do you understand now that there is NO standard other than your own.

KITCHEN

Let's leave the bathroom and enter the kitchen. There are very few kitchens that are designed for wheelchair users. The problems are that the counter tops are about 6 to 8 inches too high. There is no way to wheel up to the sink (at any height) unless all cabinet space is taken from under the sink to make room for our legs and feet that protrude at least 24 to 30 inches from one's stomach, depending on its size. Can you wheel up sidesaddle? Sure, but expect the biggest backache of your life to be the result of having to twist your body 90 degrees for any length of time. It is the same with the range, as it is too high for safety. It also must be approached sidesaddle as well as the sink because there is no leg/foot room beneath.

The high and unsafe range problem is more easily solved than the inconvenient sink height. You can install what is called a "drop-in" range top that has no oven below and can be lowered. They also have "stick-in" ovens for cabinet installations that can be installed any distance from the floor for safe use for us sitters. Keep in mind that persons who are at highest risk of accidents are those of us who have any impairment in our standing or walking and/or with the use of only one hand/arm, and those who are paralyzed and in scooter or wheelchair who have little or no balance.

The problem with lowering the sink is that all too often the waste- or sewer-line opening into the wall is too high (water doesn't run uphill.) Here again you will be calling a plumber, doing it yourself, or utilizing the knowledge and experience of a neighbor, relative, or friend. Know that in this case you are talking BIG bucks or Big work. Unlike a high kitchen range, a high sink isn't particularly dangerous; but it is certainly inconvenient.

It also makes a difference what is expected of those of us with disabilities and for how long it will be expected of us. If you are renovating either kitchen or bath, it makes a difference if the person for whom this renovation is taking place is 20 or 80 years of age. If your loved one is 20 years of age and you expect that person to live in your home for another 20-40 years, it is a different picture than what you would do in a situation in which that person would be living in that situation for 3-10 years. Everyone must decide for himself just what priorities should be placed on renovation. Also keep in mind that it doesn't take much to use up $3,000 to $10,000 in costs for kitchen or bath remodeling.

Floor Covering

And finally, what about those thick, plushy, almost-impossible-to-roll-on carpets. Well, get rid of them as soon as it is within your means. You will soon learn that it takes quite an effort to move on them whether you are the person in the wheelchair trying to push your own chair or you are the family member who is trying to push us with or without our help. Those of us who are forced to shuffle, use a cane or walker also have a difficult time overcoming the friction of plush/ padded carpet. When you shop for carpet find a low pile, hard backed carpet (commercial grade if possible).

Demand direct glue-down to the floor without pad. If the company or installer refuses to lay carpet without a pad, call the manufacturer, explain your situation, and ask their opinion. If the manufacturer agrees with the carpet company and/or installer, then either get a different carpet or a different installer, or both. Any pad, even a thin one, will defeat the purpose. It is standard procedure to tell you the carpet won't wear well without a pad and that to protect your investment you must install one. Heiferdust, I have used carpets without padding for 35 years with no problem.

However, if you drop a heavy, sharp object on the carpet without a pad, it will cut easier than one with pad. If that happens it can be repaired either with adhesive or patching it with a piece of carpet scrap that you should always collect from the carpet layer. The more scrap you saved the better in case of having to match pattern.

Now let's get away from the house architecture and on to the furniture and other interior decorations. In my counseling I always stress the importance for families to help make the limited member as independent as possible. This may mean a special electric hospital bed, a power wheelchair, lower/higher tables or other altered furniture, or rearranged furniture. Train family and friends to push in chairs, pick up shoes, etc.—anything that might be in the way.

A quick browse through most medical supply companies will astound you as to the availability of self-help devices. If you ask me what I despise most about my disability it is when I am forced to ask for help, and most of us with disabilities feel the same way. Please arrange lamps and furniture so we can get around easily. It may mean placing a few items in storage. I have been in the homes where even though a family member was in a wheelchair, I had to pick my way through the house as one would pick his way through a chicken yard. And you can't fully understand that if you have never tried to maneuver a wheelchair through a chicken yard and avoid the chicken pfbbt.

Anything we can safely do for ourselves will cause less stress and demands on the person who must otherwise do it for us. Not only that, but it will give us a much better sense of self-worth and it will minimize our limitations rather than being constantly confronted with misery of knowing that we can't, we Can't, we CAN'T. In today's world there are devices to do just about everything we are unable to do for ourselves.

There are devices for persons who can only use one hand for a task that needs two hands. There is velcro to take the place of buttons, zippers, and shoe laces. There are electronic devices that turn appliances on and off. Reach extenders are available like in the old days when the grocer needed to get an item on a high shelf. We now have dogs trained to help us. Bless the computer, and for a mind and the ability to press a single key that can set in motion just about any schedule we want and can afford.

Ah, that's the tough word right there—afford. All these things cost money and most of us who ever had any have spent all ours on our hospital and rehabilitation stays. Know that this is a great day in which to have a disability, but that we must use our heads as to the priorities of problems and solutions. Spend wisely! Think ahead!

Environmental Barriers

Then there are environmental barriers. Man made the architectural ones and God made the ones in our environment. They are anything over or through which a person with a particular limitation cannot navigate easily: sandy beaches, hills, mountains, woods, etc. Some of this can be changed and some is beyond sensible restructuring.

The National Parks have done a great job in making many of the spots of beauty accessible. The North Rim of the Grand Canyon is much less used than the South Rim, so it was surprising to discover they had several wheelchair paths and a special elevator for persons with disabilities that allowed access to the lower vista. There are many publications regarding accessibly in the National Parks, cities, and historical places of interest. Write or call the Agencies or Chambers of Commerce. You will be surprised what has opened up to you.

Since so much is happening in the area of accessibility because of the Americans with Disabilities Act, any accessibility list that could be printed at any given time would be obsolete before the presses had stopped rolling. *ANY* place you wish to go, write or call regarding possible accommodations for persons with disabilities. State your needs or what you cannot do to make sure they understand your disability.

One time special arrangements were made for being preloaded at the airport, and when I arrived at the gate the attendant expected me to get up out my wheelchair and somehow walk to my seat. She said with a tinge of disgust, "You should have told us you couldn't walk." My reply was "Lady, if I could walk I wouldn't be in this wheelchair." What had escaped me is that some persons use a wheelchair for convenience. At the time of the arrangements the airline personnel should have asked me if I was able to walk onto the plane or down the aisle.

Also be prepared for some "strange" accommodations in the name of accessibility. Too many times we have arrived at a motel where reservations had been made for wheelchair accommodations only to discover 1) an employee overlooked the wheelchair designation on the reservation, 2) the motel management foolishly promised the non-disabled occupants of the previous day that they could have *that* room for another night, the accessible one which had been assigned to us for that night, and 3) the "accessible" room assigned was up four steps.

In the case of number #1, the management routed out some non-disabled person from a "handicapped" room and asked them to move to another room. Everyone involved was unhappy. In case #2 they grudgingly let us occupy a regular room that was being remodeled. In case #3 they called around and found us an accessible room in another motel at 10 p.m. And there have been many more almost disasters.

What we must keep in mind in all of these inquests and arrangements is that the able-bodied world does not have the same definition of *accessible*. This is why it is so important to communicate our individual requirements. Sometimes I have followed up the reservation with a letter, and sometimes with a last-minute call if the reservation was made several days or weeks before we arrive.

Hopefully, these shared experiences of mine and others will help motivate you to look at your situation with challenge rather than despair.

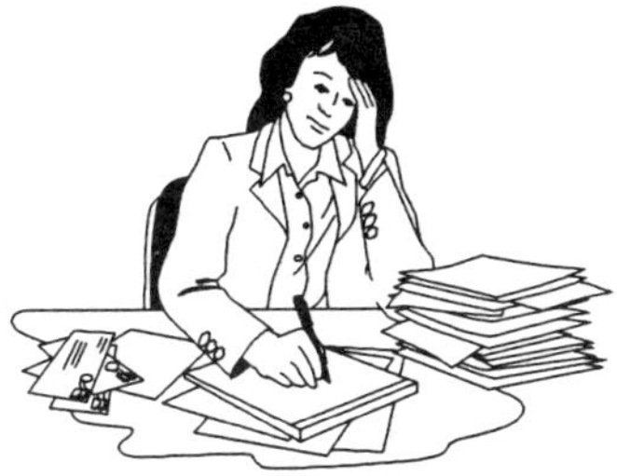

Chapter 6

Managing Stress and Anger

WHAT IS STRESS?

We all talk about it, but what is it and what does it do to us? The place to find a definition that has to do with our minds and bodies is in the dictionary: "any stimulus, as fear or pain, that disturbs or interferes with the normal physiological equilibrium of an organism." So now we know what stress is—or do we?

The best definition I can come up with is that anything (usually negative or worrisome) to which your mind travels the moment you put it in neutral is stress. Keep in mind there is such a thing as happy stress caused by doing happy things. We need happy stress to keep us from becoming lumps of clay. An example of happy stress is the flurry of stress-related activities that evolve from preparing for a party or having out-of-town guests whom you are anxious to see. If you view the end results of the stress as happy, it is positive stress—if an unhappy ending is anticipated, it is negative stress.

The problem is that what is stress for some may not be stress for others. Not only is their stress unique, some have less of it. Some folks as we say, are so laid back that few things in life cause them stress. Some of us are always in a dither about something.

To me, not having money in the checking account the day a bill is due would be very stressful. Having car trouble is stressful. Being late for anything is stressful. Feeling that I have more to do than I have time in which to do it is stressful. Some of you agree and some of you chuckle. I know persons who could have a pile of bills with no money and it doesn't bother them a bit. Who worries about being late? Who worries about car trouble? My son-in-law does and he's a mechanic.

What I want you to realize is that we each have our own bag of stress, and what is stress for one person can be a delightful challenge to another.

Let's not forget the uniqueness of stress as related to the uniqueness of personality. Actually, it is personality that dictates the type and level of psychological/emotional stress in our lives. I am one of a kind; you are one of a kind, just like a snowflake. Therefore, your stress and my stress is unique to each of us—it is one of a kind.

So how do we think we can take a stress management course and come up with a universal approach to a unique problem? I have a difficult time keeping a smug smile off my face when someone tells me that they have paid or are going to pay money to learn how to manage stress. Too often the person who has taken a course or attended a seminar comes away feeling that he or she really has a handle on coping with stress. Unless you practice what has been preached, you have just learned some new words and new ways of verbalizing your stress. From a functional position, nothing much has changed except your vocabulary. Now I am in trouble with all the professional stress-management people.

Well, are there some universal practices that work when applied to a unique problem that is causing stress? Yes, if we make the correct diagnosis of what is *causing* the stress and a proper application of a principle. On one list of stress-reducing behavior was the suggestion to "dance nude in front of your pets." However, after your pets have recovered from the shock and you perhaps have reduced your stress for the moment, if you have not done anything to reduce the *cause* of the stress, your pets are in for another performance.

In my seminars with persons newly diagnosed with multiple sclerosis, coping with stress is one of the topics. Following is a list of thirty suggestions that I have collected, mostly from unremembered sources. Some will fit your situation and some won't.

1. Accept what you cannot change.
2. If your disability allows it, get up a little earlier each morning.
3. Don't rely on your memory. Write things down.
4. Do unpleasant tasks as soon as possible.
5. Procrastination is a common cause of stress. DO IT NOW!
6. Be prepared to wait.

7. Dwell on the positive and your zest for life will return.
8. Keep things simple. Don't complicate your life with frills.
9. Avoid those who worry and/or complain.
10. Organize yourself, don't just talk about it.
11. Be more flexible.
12. Eliminate negative self-talk.
13. Do only one thing at a time.
14. Delegate to responsible people and forget it.
15. Learn to relax.
16. Learn to forgive.
17. Plan ahead. Don't let your gas tank get below ¼ full.
18. Know where your responsibilities end and another's begin.
19. Do not repress your feelings.
20. Express your feelings to someone you trust.
21. Seek support when the need arises.
22. Discard or repair things that don't work properly.
23. Allow yourself time to grieve over your losses.
24. Live in the present and leave yesterday behind.
25. Like in poker, know when to fold.
26. Quit blaming yourself (or others).
27. Keep special or sacred memories close to your heart.
28. Manage your energy well. Have sensible energy priorities.
29. Pick up the pieces of your life and slowly put them back together but know that life can never be the same.
30. Take good care of you health; focus on survival and hope for the future.

Can We Always Recognize Stress?

One of the strange aspects of stress is that more often than not it goes undetected. In a psychology class in which we were studying the effects of stress on the digestive system, we had a film showing a cat whose digestive system was exposed. It was fascinating to watch the peristaltic action process of the stomach. The cat was locally anesthetized and relaxed, but it was alert to its surroundings. It was on a comfortable table in a room approximately the size of a regulation basketball court. Quietly a dog was brought in on a leash at the very furthest corner and made to lie down and not move or bark. The moment the dog entered the large room, the cat's digestive process stopped cold although the cat appear nonchalant. There were no other signs that the dog was upsetting the cat. Immediately upon the removal of the dog, the cat's stomach began to churn again.

What does that say to us? It says more than a dog in a cat's presence stops digestion. It tells us the cause of some of our indigestion. It tells us the results of threatening behavior at mealtime for children. It tells us that although we may appear normal to ourselves and others, something can eat away at our innards. If something can stop our digestion system it can cause considerable upset in other parts of our body.

Animals and humans have what is termed survival behavior. When sensing danger, the procedure begins with an alert/alarm response and climaxes with the decision to face it or run (flight or fight). The adrenalin gland squirts out a small, measured amount of its chemical to bring the body and mind to wake up to the possible danger. If this danger is perceived to becoming more threatening, more adrenalin is pumped into the system. The attack mode is the peak of this response to danger. Humans and animals can perform unbelievable mental and physical feats in the "attack" mode. Parents have been known to lift cars off their children. Have you ever done something in a time of stress and later wondered how you ever managed to do it?

What Damage Can Stress Do To Our Bodies?

Even in a simple alert mode, the body is being energized by greater-than-normal amounts of chemicals (not only adrenalin). It is like racing our automobile engine in preparation for a good start in a race. But what if the engine is raced for many hours? or days? or months? or years? Well, you say, "It's hard on it and you will shorten its life." Right! And so it is with our health when we are racing our engines. If we are under known or unknown stress, our body chemistry changes and we are racing our engines and it will shorten our lives.

We have a great and wonderful auto-immune system that wards off bacteria and other enemies. Recent studies have linked stress to a repression of our auto-immune system thereby making us more vulnerable to attack from sickness and disease. Back in the late fifties, Dr. Hans Selye, a Canadian researcher proposed the theory that stress was the cause of *all* sickness. Of course he was the laughing stock of the medical community. However, his experiment with rats at least gave evidence that *some* illnesses were stress related, and I am not sure he isn't about 90% correct.

One of the experiments used two groups of rats: the control group and the experimental group. The food and environment of both groups were identical, but the experimental group was given a slight electrical shock that did no more than to make the rats periodically uncomfortable for a fraction of a second (a slight tingling in their feet). After several weeks applying what is called a "noxious stimulant," both the control and the experimental groups were chilled by allowing them to swim in icy water for a short time. Of course the groups were continuously kept separate or the study would be of no value. Interestingly, all—100%—of the rats who had received the bothersome electrical shock came down with colds—rat colds, I suppose. None of the non-stressed control group became ill.

Although no one has brought forth empirical evidence to prove or disprove the theory that stress causes *all* ills, we know it adversely affects our health. Most of us recognize in our own lives that when we are stressed out, this is when we often contract colds or are invaded by a virus. Every man in the polio ward whom I had opportunity to know was under some sort of stress at the time the polio virus made its attack. Stress had reduced the auto-immune system to a point where it was too weak to fight the virus. Reduce stress and live happier and longer. It has become common knowledge that cancer, AIDS, multiple sclerosis are all disorders of the auto-immune system.

Of course we know that no one lives a stress-free life. However, we should attempt to keep it at a minimum by using whatever method works for us—mind over matter, or drug over mind.

Is Stress Additive?

What do we mean, is stress additive? Simply that each individual stress is added to the other stresses we are carrying. This is what happens when we say, "I have had a rotten day." What made it rotten? A power failure occurred and the alarm didn't go off. You went to leave for work or play and the car had a flat tire. Oh, you ran out of gas. The seam on the new dress ripped. You forgot your lunch, and on an on we could go. Our reaction to stress is not on an individual basis but all the stresses added together. If one morning your alarm failed to wake you, a flat tire greeted you in the garage, and because of your stress you ran out of gas, each one of these things combined with the others—and the office secretary asked you a simple question and you exploded.

To understand the importance of individual stresses adding themselves together for a total weight, you must also understand that each of us has our own threshold or container for stress. My stress bucket might be a quart; yours might be a gallon. No matter what it measures, it is individually ours, and when we exceed our capacity we spill over.

Keep in mind now that we all have a stress bucket into which we toss our individual amounts of stress. Do the pennies experiment to get the idea. Take a small glass of water (think of it as your stress bucket), fill it with water to near the top and carefully slip pennies into it one at a time. At some given moment the glass will run over because you have exceeded its limit. But it was only a small, thin piece of copper that spilled the water—and so it is with stress. Add all the small stresses (pennies) together and when you exceed your limit (threshold of tolerance) you run over. By eliminating just one penny (stressful situation) you would not have had to clean up the mess. Stress in our lives is no different. Remember, it was the proverbial straw that broke the camel's back!

Let's get back to stress in our lives caused by physical or mental limitations. Any type of disability intensifies any of the stresses your personality dictates, and then adds a few more of its own. Attempting to cope with a disability, your own or another person's, will make mole hills look like mountains. When we are unable to recognize these mountains as the mole hills they really are, we react to them as we perceive them, and the stress is multiplied. Reducing hurtful stress in anyone's life is important, but because there is more of it when a disability is involved we must be militant in our war against stress.

What About Pain?

In our definition of stress, there was the word *pain*. Well, I am an organism, so how does pain affect me? We are not going to get deeply into the subject of pain, but I want you to realize its potential for causing stress which does all those nasty things to us that we just read.

The body has its own way of coping with pain. When something hurts, the brain tells the manufacturing plant to develop or release more endorphins. We can even "psych" up or induce our manufacturing plant into higher output to withstand pain by the power of thinking. I was always fascinated by the Indian fakir (not faker) who could lie on a bed of spikes and not howl with pain, or those walking on white-hot coals. The orientals use this phenomenon in their martial arts performances. If I tried to break a board with my fist, I would suffer excruciating *pain.*

Long-lasting, non-treatable pain is devastating to the body and mind, even what is often referred to as a "nagging" back ache. In the past decade there has been much work done on treating pain by all sorts of methods including bio-feedback. There are pain clinics and pain centers of every size and description. What none of us wants to hear is, "You'll just have to learn to live with it." However, that is just what many of us have to do.

How Can We Control Our Anger

In chapter one we talked about anger, but this was primarily related to anger over the happening of our disability. Now we are discussing anger that is generated by things other than the happening of our disability—the happenings and frustrations of daily living. You may not be disabled yourself, but you may suffer the infuriating frustrations of disability if your are deeply involved with someone who is. You are human, and therefore you must cope with one of our most volatile human emotions.

Those of us with disabilities have the added dimension of our limitations. A number of years ago in a seminar I was the speaker on disability. Several speakers overran their time limit and the five minutes each of us had been allowed for the recap was cut to one word. How could one word describe disability. Suddenly it came to me—frustration.

Of the common causes of anger, frustration (being powerless) is perhaps the most common; therefore, it would be expected that persons with disabilities will be more possessed by anger than if they were able bodied. One man said to me: "You know, if I didn't know how to do so many things, my disability would be much easier to handle." To have the mental ability to complete difficult tasks but have a body that disallows that ability, is frustrating beyond measure.

Unchecked anger is dangerous both to the person who is wielding it as well as the object or target of that anger. That object can be another human or just a *thing*. My anger is usually vented at things—things that go wrong; things that don't work right; things that are dropped or broken—things, things, things—not at people. My anger is most often directed at myself.

Anger is dangerous not only to things and others, but to you and me. However, we must differentiate between *righteous indignation* and uncontrolled fury. A slight irritation is on one end of the spectrum, and angry-enough-to-kill on the other end. Apart from the legal consequences of uncontrolled anger, there are the physical consequences. Anger and stress act very similarly on the body. Have you not heard the phrase, "hot under the collar" as another definition of anger? Yes, you actually do get hot under the collar. Why? It is because your heart rate increases, the adrenalin flows, and all the other stress-related changes that take place.

There are myriads of books written on coping with anger, but you may not have read or owned any of them. This book you are reading so it is my responsibility to give you some of my solutions for coping with anger.

Unfortunately, we are sometimes victims of our ancestors or ethnic backgrounds. Some ethnic groups are noted for their "short fuses," and most often are very proud of that fact. In some families anger out of control is tolerated, in others it is not. Anger-aroused physical attacks are acceptable in some cultures, in others they are not.

The old steam locomotive required a "head of steam" to move. A "working head of steam" was needed to allow the locomotive to do what it was designed to do—work. And finally, the "dangerous head of steam" that could rupture the boiler or tubes. *The Wreck of the Old Southern 97*, the song of the prior century, told the story of the disaster of a dangerous head of steam. Of course in later years safety valves were installed on steam boilers to prevent such explosions.

Our "working head of steam" is important for living life, but we must guard against the danger of having too much of a good thing. For a few more words on anger and wrath, let's turn to the oldest book on psychology that I have in my library—the *Bible*. Anger is mentioned 260 times, angry 69 times, and wrath 214 times. Can we gather value and advice on handling anger from these verses?

"He that is slow to wrath is of great understanding: but he that is hasty of spirit exalteth folly." (Proverbs 14:29) An application of this to what we are saying is that long fuse is wise and a short fuse causes us to do or say foolish things.

"Scornful men bring a city into a snare: but wise men turn away wrath." (Proverbs 29:8) Wrathful anger of a few often puts a noose around the necks of everyone in the group .

"Be ye angry, and sin not: let not the sun go down upon your wrath." (Ephesians 4:26) There is nothing wrong with anger if it is held in check, but don't let it fester and create an open wound. The key to this is forgiveness (#16 in the list of stress-management practices)—and the sooner, the better. Forgive others and yourself.

Okay, but what is the most used weapon against anger that I use myself and encourage others to use it? It is the act of "nipping it (the anger) in the bud." Before the working head of steam gets out of hand, do something about it. STOP! ANALYZE what is happening or going to happen. Then search for some way to help you cool off and let the scalding steam pass out safely. Do something else for a while. Get a cup of coffee. Do something the moment you feel the pressure rising. Once your pop valve opens, you can't shut it off.

There is nothing we have discussed on anger that is unusual or profound. You knew all this, but you may not have realized how disability exacerbates or adds to normal run-of-the-mill frustration. You also may not have realized that from the standpoint of body chemistry, anger and stress cause parallel reactions. Avoid negative stress and negative anger and you will live happier, healthier, and longer.

Also keep in mind that persons with brain dysfunctions, depressed or otherwise-stressed persons, often suffer a loss of emotional control. This is often the case with persons with multiple sclerosis, stroke victims, and other diseases or conditions of the nervous system. You cry more easily; you give up (or in) more easily; your anger is kindled at a lower temperature (short fuse syndrome). Reduce your level of stress and you automatically lengthen the fuse on your anger. Easier said than done, but work on controlling it for your own benefit.

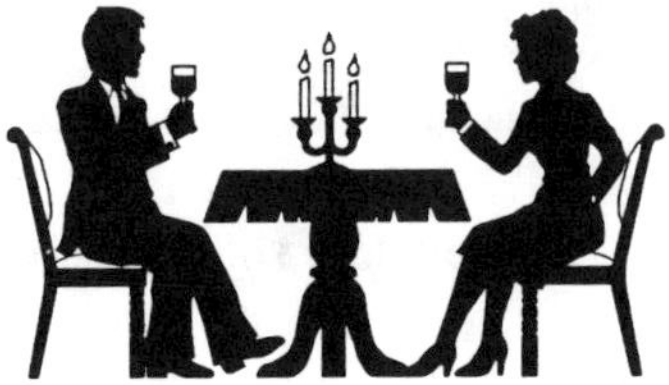

Chapter 7

Married Couples

THE STRESS OF DISABILITY IN MARRIAGE

The institution of marriage suffers from the buffeting of the waves in the "Sea of Life." It is a fragile frigate whose strength depends on what materials were used in construction, the quality of construction, the size and frequency of the waves and swells it must withstand.

A ship cannot be expected to hold up from the sea's battering if materials are used that fight each other—materials that have extremely different degrees of strength and flexibility. Marriages, like ships must have a degree of flexibility or they will rupture from the stress. In the days of wooden ships, it was when the ship stopped creaking (flexing) that the crew became alarmed. A ship must either flex and survive or be rigid and break.

What makes for a flexible marriage? It is two persons united in marriage that are willing to "creak" together. The key word is compromise. In my early theological training we were taught that compromise was evil. Whether this was meant to apply only to theological positions or not, I don't know. Unfortunately, I carried it over into all of life believing as I had been taught that compromise was a symptom of weakness. Experience has since taught me that compromise can truly be a symptom of strength when used from a position of power. That means that when the person who has the ultimate power is willing to compromise with the person with less power, it then becomes a symptom of strength.

An example of this is when I enclosed our patio. The electrical inspector gave my work the once-over, gave me a look and said, "You know, I could make you put in a receptacle *there*, but I can see that it would be very difficult and you really don't need it." That was compromise on his part from a position of power. He had total power.

It never ceases to amaze me how some people use the rule book as a bible rather than a guideline. Recently here in Arizona some endangered species of saguaro cacti were found on a man's property. He could not prove they were obtained legally and the State Department of Agriculture wanted to transplant them to public land. Most botanists were skeptical of the success of the transplant. In other words, these rare cacti would most likely die. The wise and sensible person would say, "Let them stay where they are and live." However, the little snit bureaucrat (whose salary is paid by the public) said about the fate of the saguaros, "It is a matter of principle," she said. "We want people to know we are going to enforce the law." If there is ever a person to fear it is he who cannot or will not compromise, be it an agricultural bureaucrat, a building inspector, a judge, a policeman, *or* a spouse.

Persons of this persuasion who have the power but are unwilling to compromise usually do so from a position of weakness—a personal weakness. Weakness or fear dictates no compromise because compromise invites criticism. Weak people cannot withstand criticism. Find an uncompromising person no matter who or what degree of power they possess, and you will find him or her to be an internally-weak person.

Flexibility In Marriage

When we talk about flexibility in marriage, just what do we mean by flexible? Well, just exactly what you think it means: the opposite of being rigid or unmovable. Rigid thoughts and ideas break under pressure just like ships. It is flexibility that absorbs much of the tug and grunt with interpersonal relationships, whether it is working on a committee or coping with marriage.

Most of the unhappiness that is generated in today's marriages is because of unwillingness to bend. Each of us entered our marriage union with a preconceived idea of what it should be. Why are 50% of today's marriages now ending in divorce? One reason is that much more thought is being given to what you will get than what you give.

In most discussion groups or counseling sessions, one of the first questions you are told to ask yourself is, "What do I want out of this relationship?" That's a good start, but only a start. It must be balanced with an equally soul-searching question, "What do I expect to give to this union?" Learn to communicate: talk openly with one another.

Partnerships, of which marriage is the most intimate and hopefully long lasting, have much in common. Business partnerships and marriage have inherent strengths and weaknesses. They also have dogged problems, one of worst being when one partner is felt to not be carrying his or her part of the load. My father went into a linotype business partnership in 1928. Although his and his partner's skills were very complementary, they had one big problem—liquor. Every time the shop became overloaded with work, his partner would go on a drunk for several days. Needless to say, the partnership didn't last.

Sometimes these inequalities are just perceived and some times they are real. When looking at perceived notions it reminds me of when we look at teenager's love and call it "puppy love," meaning that it has no depth. Well, to the puppies it certainly has all the dimensions of adult love. We might just as well realize right now that to persons who perceive something, to them it is real until proven otherwise. Very often that proof is difficult.

This is also true with perceived ideas of a marriage partner who is limited by some physical, intellectual, or emotional disability. What can or can't they do? Somewhere during these past few decades we have taught as gospel truth that you can achieve *any* goal you select if you put enough of yourself into it. What we forget is that all of us—*all of us*—run out of ourselves. We all have limitations, some more, some less. When we come to the end of our rope there is no amount of drive that can push us beyond it. No, all goals are not attainable to all people, with or without a disability, no matter how hard we try. A disability in any form or shape further limits our ability to achieve our goals.

The most distressing thing I see is persons who do not know or cannot see their limitations. The natural result is anger and frustration. It is difficult enough to attempt to cope with the truth, but it is impossible to even set realistic goals if you are unaware of your limitations. To set an unrealistic goal is to invite inevitable failure. Failure is the seed of self-depreciation that can ultimately lead to thoughts of suicide. If I fail, I am worthless. If I am worthless I am a drag on those I love. If I am a drag on my loved ones, the kindest and most loving thing I can do for them is to remove myself from this earth. Add a disability to the most solid marriage and there is the possibility of deep trouble.

Hard-hat Areas In Marriage

Let's look at some of the areas that seem to house a time bomb. The first is loss of freedom. Of course there is no such thing in marriage or business in which one does not lose freedom. However, the loss of freedom must be equal for each partner.

In your childhood did you have a turtle for a pet? Do you remember how frantic it became if you pinned it to the ground and kept it from moving? It put every ounce of (super-turtle) strength into trying to lift itself off the ground and get loose from whatever it was that was holding it. That is a survival mechanism for the turtle. It if cannot get free it will die. Of course in the case of our pet, we only held it captive for a few moments.

We humans are like that in some ways. If our freedom is taken away, our survival instincts take over. Apart from our constitutional rights, who can rob us of our freedom? Our spouse, for one, can unknowingly or knowingly usurp our power. Today's woman is not as willing to give up her freedom in marriage to be *managed* by her spouse. She kicks and screams when she is shunted to the sideline. But what if a disability is injected and she cannot "kick and scream" anymore? There are some women (and in some cases, men) who had equal input into their partnership until disability or illness came along. When your opinions are no longer taken seriously, no one allows you to make a decision for others in the family or even yourself, the time bomb is about to explode.

Money is another area of danger. Some have erroneously quoted the *Bible* as saying that money is the root of all evil. It doesn't say that; it reads that "*the love of money is the root of all evil.*" Regardless, money is at the root of better than 50% of marriage problems. When you add a disability you also add medical expenses and often the loss of a second income. One must then either find additional income or cut back on the style of living. Neither is easy.

It was originally my intention to do a short chapter on money management, but it is my opinion that you either have the skill of managing money or you do not. It is not something that is learned. Oh, it is possible to hone a skill, but like many other skills it must be there in the first place. On several occasions in group work we discussed this topic. When I laid out a budget for them, it was met with sneers and sarcasm. One woman snorted, "I won't live like that!." Well, you will if you have only enough money to live at that level. Unfortunately, so many just look around and think that everyone should be able to afford the same style of living. After all, isn't that part of *The Great American Dream*? Face it! That is a dream and only a dream, and if you overspend it becomes a nightmare.

Money management is simply a management of your financial resources. Do not spend more than you make—in fact, spend a little less so there will be some savings. My children were told from childhood that if they were not putting something away out of each allowance they were actually going backwards. Once you realize that neither you (nor the federal or local government) can continuously spend more than is taken in, you have the simple formula to keep you out of BIG trouble. But of course the formula must be religiously applied. The key words are discipline and priorities. On occasion I counsel a family who has gotten itself into a financial bind through credit buying, and they are smart enough to cut up their plastic money and pay cash for everything except automobiles and homes. Wise persons buy what they can afford; the foolish buy what they want even when it is beyond their means.

My list of priorities will not be yours, and yours will not be mine. Let's leave money for a paragraph and look at food. I love to look at food and it loves to look at me. Every pound of weight gained I must lift in and out of the car, in and out of bed, on and off the toilet, and wheel it wherever I go. When I look at food and the saliva begins to flow, I must set a priority: do I want to enjoy that food or do I want to be mobile. Do I want to have a good taste in my mouth for a few minutes or do I want to be able to move without help. It is my choice and it is my priority. After actual necessities, all spending should be prioritized, whether it is *spending* calories or dollars.

We don't expect children to have sensible priorities in much of anything from spending their allowance to spending their time. That comes with experience and growing into adulthood. Unfortunately, some of us never leave childhood. The socio-psychological tool for assessing maturity is the ability of the person to postpone gratification. That's where the statement originated, "Animals and children want it *NOW*." With that statement, rate your maturity.

Most people fall into two general categories—today people and tomorrow people, spenders and savers, borrowers and loaners, throwers and salvagers, disciplined and undisciplined. Often the undisciplined appear to be undisciplined not only in their spending habits, but also in food and drug consumption, in time management, and in most other areas of living. Know your strengths and weaknesses. If you are one of the undisciplined, it may be your good fortune to be married to one who isn't. Be smart and turn over the money management to the partner best equipped for it, and gender is not a factor. That's all for money.

Talk about frustrations in a marriage, how about anger? If a family is forced to cut back on their living standard because one of the family member becomes disabled, it is not uncommon for family members to get angry. Do they vent their anger at the disability? No, it is all too often directed toward the innocent one, the person with the disability. And sometimes the disabled one vents anger on the innocent non-disabled mate. The classic textbook example of "misplaced aggression" can be seen here and in the story of the parents who complained to the school board about a discipline problem with their son. The school board crabbed at the superintendent, who in turn chewed on the principle. The principal called in the teacher who then pounced on the child, who in turn went home and kicked the dog. After all, how does one "kick" a disability.

One of the most common complaints is that the non-disabled spouse does not understand us, and sometimes it seems that they don't even want to try to understand. First of all, if you are expecting your non-disabled spouse to understand you, your feelings, your limitations, your disability, et al, forget it. They won't because they can't. As well as my wife knows me since we were kids in grade school, and has been married to me for 44 years, she cannot participate in my innermost feeling about my disability. What you have not experienced you can never *fully* understand—neither you nor I. What we can expect is that each of us will try to understand our mate. Then accept our mate's limited degree of understanding us as well as our own limited understanding of them.

When marriage and disability are discussed in individual or group counseling, the subject of divorce seems to pop up almost immediately. Does it mean an end to the marriage? The following three reprinted magazine articles should help answer that question.

Reprinted by Permission: *ACCENT ON LIVING* magazine, Fall-1991

Does Disability Mean Divorce?

Timing, duration and tightness of a relationship determine if it can survive

by Robert Lovering

With teeth clenched, the wife of a newly-disabled husband growled, "If I had wanted to be a nurse, I would have gone to nursing school." At that moment I was a bit surprised even though I had been a psychological counselor specializing in disability for more than twenty years. It was not her dislike for so-called nursing duties to her "thirty-something" husband that startled me, but her honesty and vehemence concerning these duties that had been thrust upon her. With the onset of disability, this marriage relationship had taken a sharp twist.

Of all our personal relationships, the most potentially intimate and therefore most fragile is that of marriage or living together WOBC (without benefit of clergy). In a society in which approximately half of marriages end in divorce, complicate this with a disability and what hope is there for a relationship to endure, to say nothing about being happy and rewarding?

I am often asked if relationships that include a disability fall into any types of distinguishable categories. My experience which is now closing in on forty years says, "Yes." The first category is related to the timing of the disability in a relationship. The second is related to the duration of the relationship before disability. The third is the tightness of the relationship bond before disability became a factor.

The timing of the disability is important. Did the relationship begin with two physically-able persons, or with one or both having a disability? In a recent counseling session the young husband looked at me and said, "I want out; I want a wife with whom I can hike, ski, and be athletically competitive." If the disability was known and understood prior to beginning the relationship, generally the ground is much more firm. Shaky ground occurs when a disability is injected into a mature relationship. A disability does not have to fracture a marriage, but it will certainly change it. My wife married me, wheelchair and all. Of course there were some surprises in our marriage as in all developing intimate relationships, but my disability was not one of them.

Generally, one would think the longer the marriage the greater its strength, but duration does not indicate strength. Many relationships are held together by a thread and may last many years if there are no traumas. A disability is like an acid that eats away the veneer and exposes the nature of our true self; likewise, a disability exposes a relationship for what it is. In most cases in which disability may appear to be the culprit, it could just as easily have been some other "straw that broke the camel's back."

There is no way to measure the "glue" or strength of either a wood or metal joint or a personal relationship until it is tested.

There is no way to know the breaking point of either until it shatters. In personal relationships it is not the duration but the individual commitment that counts. Commitment cannot be measured; it can only be observed in conduct.

Finally, can we expect a wholesomeness in a relationship in which a disability is inserted that seemingly forces one to be a "servant" of the other? My answer is, "Yes," because I have seen it in my own marriage and many others in which a spouse was disabled—before, after, or otherwise. The problems that I see are usually not because of what the disabled mate can't do; it is more often what the able-bodied mate feels the disabled one could do and doesn't. Isn't that true of any relationship? We expect our business or marriage partner to carry their share of the work. When we don't carry our end of the plank, trouble brews.

When I do everything of which I am capable, our marriage hits no snags. I don't demand or expect my wife to do all she does for me. Those extra things she does are out of love—I appreciate them and I tell her.

Reprinted by Permission: *ACCENT on living* magazine, Summer-1992

Marriage To Quad Ends In Divorce

by Shelli Ivie

Could this marriage have been saved?

What would you have done in this situation?

After reading Susie Blackmun's article, "For better or for Worse" in the Winter issue of *ACCENT*, I felt compelled to write about my marriage to a quad. My husband and I had been dating for nine months when he was involved in a drunk-driving accident in which he was a passenger. That fateful night left him paralyzed from the chest down. He was diagnosed as a C¾ quad with no hope of regaining any functional use of his arms or hands. One year later we were married.

I was 23-years old and had fantasies of white picket fences and happily ever afters, not uncommon for most young brides. Even though I understood the seriousness of his condition and his limitations, it didn't matter—we were in love. Love is that all-encompassing concept that deflects any negativity or grasp of reality.

I was truly content and happy with my life. I was married to the man I loved, we had a nice home, and we were fortunate enough to have enough money to live comfortably without me having to go to work.

It sounds picture perfect, doesn't it? There was just one problem—I ceased to exist. I became my husband's arms and legs. I was his extension to the rest of the world and exchanged my role as wife for that of care giver.

I was warned by many professionals to not fall into the trap of care giver. They said I would suffer from some abstract phenomena called burn-out, but in spite of their warnings, I was determined to do it all, become a superwoman. I refused to let anyone else care for my husband—I felt it was my duty as his wife.

Anyone who has lived with or cared for a disabled spouse or loved one knows what a demanding and stressful job it can be. Spouses who become the main care giver are nothing short of wizards. They schedule, organize and juggle their lives around the disabled person. Every day is a balancing act while they try to manage the house and second guess their spouses needs while neglecting their own.

Suzie wrote in her "For Better or Worse" article, "Care givers often assume so much responsibility that they cease having a life of their own. And, "Those care givers who sacrifice everything for the needs of their husbands or wives often end up living in a cocoon of despair."

After living in a wave of despair for several months of full-time care giving, I realized I needed some help. The insurance company would pay for two hours a day of care by an R.N. I decided to have the nurse help me in the mornings which were the most stressful time of the day. By then, my husband had become so dependent on me that he had a hard time letting anyone else help with the more personal things like bowel programs and catheterization.

Therefore without realizing it, I had set myself up for burn-out. As time went by I tried to break away and work part time. It never lasted very long though because the guilt would set in and I felt like a terrible person for leaving him with a stranger. Other problems arose also. He developed a pressure sore and was confined to bed for a couple of months. At that time I quit my job and returned home because I felt that I could care for him better than anyone else.

I found myself becoming more resentful of his disability and misplaced my anger onto him as if it were his fault that he couldn't move. We were both frustrated and angry with one another most of the time. He was angry with me because I could walk and I was angry with him because he couldn't. Our marriage had turned into a mud-slinging contest with no winners. My husband became more demanding and I fell deeper into a depressed state.

After five years of sleepless nights and endless demands on my time, I became so burned out that I ran away and I never went back. Anyone who has been through a divorce knows how painful it can be. The feelings of loss and guilt that accompany a failed marriage are overwhelming. We often reflect on what went wrong and why and what-ifs. I think it's a normal feeling and one that needs to be explored in order to learn and grow from our mistakes.

Marriage in general is difficult and requires patience, compromise, devotion and most importantly, communication. However, when a couple has special problems to deal with because one spouse is disabled, it is doubly difficult.

In reflection I can see why our marriage didn't work. I made the biggest mistake that anyone can make when married to a disabled spouse—I became the care giver rather than the wife. Certainly becoming the full-time care giver was not the only problem that contributed to our failed marriage, but it was the biggest.

I think it is only natural that a wife wants to care for her husband, but this Florence Nightingale syndrome is really a web weaved out of fear and ignorance. Although it starts out with good intent, the end result is burn-out and pain for all involved. I only wish I had listened to others who warned me of its dangers.

I share this story so others who find themselves in a similar situation may have the knowledge to learn from my mistakes. And if you are in this situation, please find help. A marriage should be a partnership where both people love and care for each other equally. It is not healthy, emotionally or physically, when one spouse in any marriage becomes totally dependent or is consumed with care giving. It is irresponsible and selfish behavior for anyone to play these types of roles. Become independent rather than dependent and your lives and marriage will flourish.

Reprinted by permission: *ACCENT on living magazine,* Fall-1992

It's Performance That Counts

Avoid the Traps That Can Cause a Marriage to Fail

by Robert Lovering

As Shelli Ivie felt compelled to write about her failed marriage, "MARRIAGE TO QUAD ENDS IN DIVORCE," so I find myself compelled to attempt to answer the two questions posed by *ACCENT*, Summer 1992: 1) Could this marriage be saved? and 2) What would you have done in this situation?

Shelli's problem is much more prevalent than commonly thought. One reason may be that few persons have the honesty and courage to vent their emotions and open themselves to criticism as Shelli did. My counseling practice of nearly 40 years (specializing in problems in which disability is a factor) currently sees better than 70% of referrals being involved in some way with marital discord resulting from a spouse being disabled.

Who knows if this marriage could have been saved? Perhaps it may have been if there had been sound, sensible premarital counsel and/or early intervention and close follow-up to escape the common pitfalls of marriage as well as the added pitfalls introduced by disability. But to whom could you or this couple turn?—look to the page after page of counselors in your Yellow Pages? or perhaps your priest, rabbi, or minister? Unfortunately, very few of these professionals are experienced or knowledgeable regarding the unique problems provoked by a disability. It is unfortunate that there is not a nationwide network of Al-anon type support groups for care givers! However, for even the wisest of counsel to be effective the persons involved must 1) recognize they have a problem, 2) desire to solve it, and 3) seek competent advice.

So with pen in hand my eyes searched this *ACCENT* article to see if there were any obvious red flags. There were more than I had expected. Of course there were those common-to-all ones such as unrealistic dreams and love-conquers-all, but then there were those unique to care giving such as lost identity, the "trap" of care giving, guilt, despair, resentfulness, endless demands, and misplaced anger.

All of the above are so common in care giving. It is unfortunate that those same professionals who advised her of burn-out didn't follow up with advice how to avoid it. Perhaps they did but it was ignored. The most simple medicine for burn-out is respite —getting away from the day-to-day responsibility of whatever it is that is burning you out—such as finding outside employment and paying for your respite. No matter how much devotion and love there is, it is humanly impossible to be tied constantly to anyone twenty-four hours a day, seven days a week without suffering burn-out. This also includes the parents of children with disabilities.

In care giving it is too easy to fall into a rut. A rut is a grave with both ends knocked out. It is caused by continuously doing the same thing over and over. So often these demands come from persons with a disability who somehow have developed the idea that the world, society, and especially their spouses owe them something for the losses caused by disability.

Therefore, the demands are deserved as a payback for what the disabled person has lost. Unreasonable and endless demands often stem from a thoughtless or thankless heart. Disability in itself breeds selfishness; the treatment or cure is for family and friends to not cave in to it. Behavior that is rewarded will continue!

My disability does not stem from a spinal-cord injury, and rather than being a quad, I am a post-polio paraplegic. I don't need care but do need assistance now and then. However, if I get a little too demanding my wife has learned to tell me sweetly to do it myself or wait until she has time. She is not my slave; she is my wife and partner, and I had better do my share of the work, mental or physical.

Marriage is a two-way street, and unless there is an agreement on the division of labor, there will be trouble.

There are many givers of total care who will agree with me as to the necessary attitude of both the care giver and the receiver of care. As long as the person receiving the care is thoughtful and thankful, this effort can be rewarding. When resentfulness begins to show it head, it is time for discussion and change. There certainly is a trap in care giving, but it can and should be avoided. Don't allow yourself to be motivated by guilt or duty.

Actually, Shelli discovered the solution to her own problem, but it was hindsight—too late to save the marriage. She gave us good advice in her final paragraphs. Perhaps it could be marriage-saving advice to some of you in the same situation. Don't abdicate your role as spouse for that of care giver. Beware of the "Florence Nightingale" syndrome. Please seek help.

What would you or I do under similar circumstances? It would be my hope that we would seek competent advice from someone who has personally been there, preferable one who has been successful in making the necessary adjustments. In this business of disability, academic credentials don't shine too brightly. Rather, as the Phillips Petroleum slogan says, "IT'S PERFORMANCE THAT COUNTS."

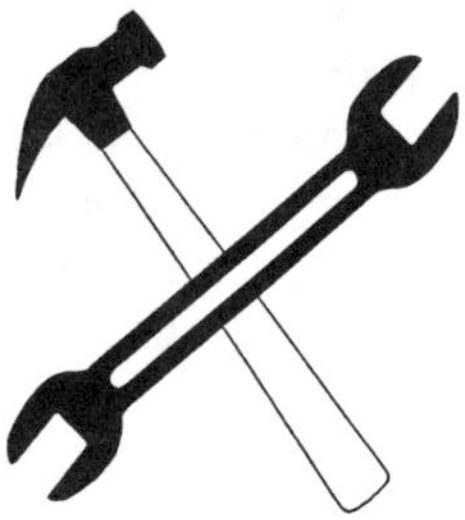

Chapter 8

TOOLS FOR EMOTIONAL COPING

DEVELOPING YOUR TOOLS

Looking at the same situation, why do some of us say we cannot cope while others of us say we can? Is it true that some can cope and others can't, or is it just a lack of trying? Are there set psychological and sociological formulas that if religiously followed will produce success in coping?

Several years ago I was invited to talk to the staff of one of our Phoenix psychiatric hospitals. The staff was made up primarily of social workers, nursing supervisors, and psychological counselors. What could I bring to them that was meaningful and different?

Over the years I had watched these same types of professional persons make the same mistake that I had made in my early years as a counselor. The mistake was best illustrated in an object lesson. Being a *tool* person it was not difficult to take one of my tool boxes and fill it with both common and uncommon tools from my workshop. As I began I am sure many wondered if this speaker had slipped a cog somewhere along the way and should really be a patient rather than an outside speaker.

My first move was to unload the tool box of all types of tools. As each tool was held up to the group they were to name it. At first it was easy: vice grips, screw driver, crescent wrench, socket wrenches, etc. Then it became more difficult: open-end crows feet, stud extractor, dial calipers, outside micrometers, inside micrometers, screw pitch gages, etc. The little or unknown tools fascinated most of the listeners. Then the lecture began.

The first question was if they thought that these tools had just been purchased at random. "No, you bought them for a specific purpose," they agreed. The next question was if they believed that the use of each tool had been mastered to the same degree. "No, it would depend upon your ability and your experience." My next question was if they had these same tools in their tool boxes at home. "Of course not!" They had admitted almost with a guffaw that their tools were different from mine. Now we were truly ready to begin the lecture.

The object lesson of the tool box was the sum and substance of the lecture. We had taken the first step and had seen that none of us had identical tools. What made us think then than all others in the world of coping with their emotions had the same set of tools? At this point we made the transfer from the mechanical tools to emotional tools.

Each of us begins to develop these behaviors and tools shortly after our departure from our mother's womb. Baby hungry—baby cry. We try something and it works. If it works once it may work twice, and so on. Baby cry—baby get fed. The other factor is our personality that works hand in hand with our experience to produce the psychological tools we most likely will use for our entire life span.

The mistake most behavior specialists make is believing that their client has the same set of psychological tools as they do. In counseling sessions we work with the persons to show them how to cope. We show off our tools from our box and try to help the persons grasp how this tool or that tool will work in their life. After the coping lesson we quiz our client on how to respond to the new methods, pick up our tools and go to the next client.

Unfortunately, when the clients are confronted by the situation on which they had been advised, they open up their box of coping tools. But alas, what they see in their box is not what the counselor showed them in the counseling session. Now what do they do?

A good counselor does not bring his tool box with him into a session. What should be done is to ask the clients to open their tool boxes to see what coping tools they have, then instruct them how to use these in *their* situation. When the session is over, the client has a new approach to using his own specially-developed tools rather than some foreign-working tool used by the counselor.

Do you see now how unique your coping skills are? What you need is advice in how to use these in your quest for coping with your emotions in time of turmoil. Examine your skills carefully. Notice some of your strengths and some of your weaknesses. Neither I nor anyone else can list your strengths and weaknesses without careful observation and/or testing.

Whatever worked for you when you were attempting to cope with emotional situation in the past will automatically (and most likely subconsciously) be tried again. Some of the general behaviors we use in coping are denial, anger, aggression, depression, diversion, eating, sleeping, drugs (prescription and non-prescription such as alcohol, tobacco, pot, etc.).

We have discussed denial in previous chapters, but we have not discussed anger as a coping tool. It becomes such when we use it to get our way. If you don't do what I ask I will blow my stack. Others conform to keep peace. Some persons, with or without a disability, use anger as a force to control others. Others threaten with aggressive or violent behavior. In these cases coping with emotional stress is accomplished by a feeling of power or control over others.

Then there are the inward "copes." Some of us simply face the problem and become depressed. Others of us find diversion by investing our minds and efforts into something else to take the edge off of our emotions. Some smoke; some "shoot up", some ingest booze; unfortunately, I eat. When I face some sort of crisis, my mind turns to my stomach, and for a few moments I have a glowing peace of mind. However, that is a lousy solution as I have to constantly lift every ounce of fat my temporary *solution* produces.

Are there not some good tools that will help us cope with stress, especially the added stress placed on our everyday lives by a disability? Yes, but there are also many bad ones. We must examine our coping tools for their effectiveness and side effects to determine which should be tossed in the garbage and which to use. It is the destructive side effects from a good drug or behavior that makes the final determination if it is a good treatment tool or a bad one.

Parallels In Coping With Stress

Most of us do not recognize coping behavior in our own lives. It just happens. More often than not, others can predict our coping behavior much better and more often that we can ourselves. When faced with stress we most often flip to "automatic pilot". When working for one of the Minneapolis health agencies, occasionally there was waiting on my desk a telephone message to return a call that I knew would be unpleasant. Immediately I began looking around my office to find some "priority" things that needed to be done first: clean my desk, check with some person about something, go to the bathroom, a few more "priority" things, and the last straw was to sharpen my pencils. When I discovered this pattern I had a good laugh at myself and set about to change that behavior.

Sometimes I could catch myself in the early throes of this unconscious procrastination. Other times I could make it last all morning. Was it mandatory that I make the call? Of course it was. Was there a way to avoid making the call? Of course not. It was my coping behavior to put off some type of unpleasant task. In a sense, I was unproductive during those times because my mind was more occupied with avoidance than solving that or any other problem. Remember #4 on page 94 in the list on coping with stress: *Do unpleasant tasks as soon as possible.*

For us to hone our coping skills or tools, we must be able to recognize them, lay them on the table, and analyze them. Sometimes you will need the help of a family member to expose your methods of coping. My wife and I have done multitudes of projects together in which neither of us could do the task alone. In my frustration with a knowledgeable mind fighting with a body that could not respond, anger became a common response and I would call myself and the innocent parts of the project all sorts of bad names. Finally, one day she had enough and walked away saying, "If you are going to do that, you can do it without my help." That cooled my heels for a time. Remember #12 on the coping-with-stress list? *Eliminate negative self talk.* Now, before I begin to ask my body to do things it cannot or should not do, I tell myself to get "realistic."

Whether it be anger, procrastination, depression, eating, or whatever, the best method to quell negative coping behavior is to "nip it in the bud." Recognize it for what it is doing or going to do to you or your relationship and take immediate measures to put a stop to it. Habits die hard, but you will find that each time you apply this new "stop" tactic to your behavior, it will soon become a habit that will be one that is positive and one you won't want to break.

GET LIFE INTO PROSPECTIVE

So many of us just seem to ride along in life and just take what comes along. All of their lives we both have told our children that one does not wait in life for things to happen: YOU MAKE THINGS HAPPEN! Prospective is another way of saying priorities. It is beyond me how one can get something into prospective without first coming to grips with priorities. List them and number them, then think of them in relationship to life—your life. As I had to give up my goal of playing the pipe organ, your disability must come into play as you reshuffle your priorities. Believe me, all priorities and goals should have a different look when one realistically factors in a disability.

We have talked some of money and time management. However, one of the key subjects of management for persons with disabilities is *energy* management. As with money and time, energy management needs priorities, and priorities yield prospective. No one has unlimited physical energy. Certainly some have more and some less, but in all of us it is limited. Unfortunately, we never seem to get much involved with priorities when there is an abundance of anything. Before polio I just went full speed ahead from the moment my feet hit the floor in the morning until my head hit the pillow at night. The limits of polio did not change my mind as it still wanted to *go*, but my body said no way.

To cope with this new limitation and frustration I had to get a new prospective on life. What really was important? How would I accomplish those goals I had decided were important? Actually, my disability did not change many of my goals in life, but it certainly changed the degree of involvement and/or success that would be achieved. How important was it for me to play basketball? An offer to play with the Rolling Gophers, a Twin Cities wheelchair basketball team, was turned down. How important was it for me to continue hunting and fishing? My hunting buddies offered to carry me to the duck blind or to sit me at the end of a cornfield for a pheasant drive. No, there were other things that now were more important in light of the energy versus value. That is what I mean by priorities. I could have played basketball or hunted, but *chose* not to do so because other things were more important to me.

Notice that nowhere has there been a suggestion that certain things *that you can do* are not important. Our list of priorities are uniquely individual and it is not my place to tell you what is important in your life. Getting your life into prospective means getting *your* life's priorities into focus. Yours and mine will be different, but they had both better be realistic in terms of money, time, and energy.

Using Diversional Tactics

There is a software disk in my drawer that is labeled, "Mind Games." One of the methods used by the computer to beat the one who foolishly challenges it is to divert the opponent's concentration to what is not important. Naturally, the computer wins.

We can develop diversional tactics in coping with emotional stress caused by a disability. If the problem cannot be solved, do not let it occupy your mind. Save your worry and your energy to be used on things that can be changed. Remember stress rule #1 on page 94: *Accept what you cannot change.*

When we begin to think negative thoughts and begin slipping into a depression, what should we do? Well, change the focus of our minds. Of course that is easier said than done, but it can be done as mentioned in chapter 1 when discussing depression. No one can control our minds without our permission, and whether we like it or not, the fact remains that we ourselves control our thoughts.

Diversion also works with worry. My mother was a worrier; I am a worrier; and my daughter is a worrier. If my wife does not arrive within a few minutes of when I think she should, my mind goes into orbit thinking of all the tragedies that have possibly befallen her. I have begged her to call me when she is going to be late, and whenever possible she does call. But those times when she can't or doesn't, my mind suffers agony until I hear the key in the door or the garage door opener. When faced with this dilemma I try to divert my thoughts to something challenging or entertaining.

The only thing diversion does is to divert our minds from something it cannot or should not be attempting to solve, or to keep us from wallowing around in forbidden psychic territory (the devil's workshop). In itself it is simply a method used to prevent a potential problem from becoming disastrous one like preventing a small grass fire from consuming the barn.

To really be sensible, we should take our diversion time and make it productive for us. Do something that needs to be done and that will lessen our stress when it is accomplished.

Occupy Your Mind

"An idle mind is the devils workshop" was an axiom often quoted by my grandmother. Not enough could be said of the therapeutic benefits of mind occupation with a hobby or some sort of challenge. Being an avid model railroader, I have been on the subscription list of *Model Railroader* magazine since the early fifties. One time there was an article by a surgeon who told how when after a surgery there were those hours of frightful waiting to see if all went well. He discovered model railroading could effectively occupy his mind during those painful waiting hours, and it worked wonders for him.

My hobbies were mostly chosen before polio, and my disability was a culling device to separate me from those I could not do, or could not do very well with my limitations. My problem was not what do I like to do, but what of my many likes is best suited to my limitations. We must choose or limit ourselves to those areas of interest that are sensible considering our limitations. Although I thoroughly enjoy old-car restoration, my body will no longer allow me to do it alone. Therefore, it must be done in conjunction with a friend who can do physically what I cannot do.

If after your disability you still have a mind left and some way to poke a keyboard, I suggest the challenge of computer operation. It may be just a mental challenge, but it also might in the end have a financial reward. It is predicted that in the years to come we are going to have more and more companies using people working at home on computers. With your home computer tied into the business computer network through what is called a telephone modem, you are as accessible to others in the corporation as you would be sitting at the next desk. The difference is that you type your communication rather than pick up a phone or turn to ask the person next to you. On the horizon I see many people in their own homes working at a computer and utilizing a fax machine.

Like so many other personality traits, more often than not it seems impossible to generate interest in hobbies or specific interest areas in those who have no interest. It appears we are born with these interests and often it will be seen in the choice of a child's toy. Would you believe that mine were toy trains, erector sets, and blocks? This one problem of mine (having too many things to occupy my mind) I wish could be passed to many of you—that of never experiencing a boring minute!

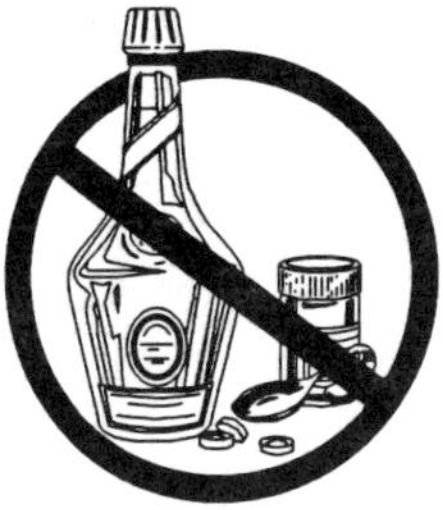

CHAPTER 9

SUICIDE CONCERNS

RELATIONSHIP OF SUICIDE AND DEPRESSION

During the last twenty years, on occasion my group work has focused on suicide. In a recent group of persons with multiple sclerosis I asked this question in this manner: "If it is embarrassing to you, don't respond, but I am interested in how many of you have fondled the idea of suicide as a solution to your problems?"

Everyone looked at the floor or some blank spot in the room to avoid the gaze of the others. One by one the hands were raised until all fifteen hands had been raised. I did not join them as I was asking the question, but in retrospect I should have. Actually, they and I were aghast. Could the thought of suicide be that prevalent among the disabled? Obviously it was.

Suicide and depression are closely related. Depression is a popular topic of discussion; unfortunately suicide is not. Rather, it seems to be a taboo subject. If it were not for the constant undertones or threats of suicide coming from persons with disabilities, we could just leave this sensitive topic alone and not get involved. Within the last year, one woman with a severe disability told me she was planning a trip to Michigan. Yes, I encouraged her, thinking of how much good it would do her to get away from it all for a week or so, and that she most likely had friends or relatives there. Then to my surprise it was discovered that she was trying to get an appointment with Dr. Kevorkian for an assisted suicide. It seems to me we had better talk about *it*.

Before we discuss suicide in relation to disability, we must first get a handle on the act itself, and then see what, if anything, is applicable to persons with disabilities. Most of us know the word means self-inflicted or intentional taking of one's life. For a death to be labeled a suicide, there must be reasonable proof of intention, the most common being a suicide note, an escape from an obvious or discovered emotional upset or trauma, or circumstances that rule out accident or foul play. This discussion of suicide is meant for the layman, not the professional sociologist, and therefore it is characterized by generalizations.

How Common Is Suicide?

Now it matters not which year or whose statistics we use, suicide is a wide-spread, frightening social problem. In my own life, I have known twice as many persons who have committed suicide as have been killed in auto accidents. These persons were neighbors, friends, relatives, and acquaintances. I have excluded from this comparison any persons who were currently or who had been at any time involved with me in counseling.

Apart from my personal experience, statistics indicate that in any fairly-current year, there will be approximately 30,000 Americans who have taken their own lives. This is only about 10% fewer than traffic fatalities. For every five accidental deaths from all causes, there will be one suicide. Then add or rearrange these statistics to reflect an unknown number of persons who are successful in making their self-inflicted death appear to be accidental, possibly for insurance purposes, sparing the family and friends from the anguish and guilt usually associated with suicide, or other reasons known only to the person himself.

When I have questioned people threatening suicide how they intended to do this, a surprising number said they planned to get in their car and accidentally-on-purpose lose control. I often see or read an account in the news media that the driver lost control and struck a bridge abutment or careened off a cliff. It makes me stop and wonder. The whole picture is staggering and frightening.

Generally, the following statements represent suicide in the United States:

1. Men kill themselves 3 to 4 times more often than women.
2. Men choose more violent means such as a knife, gun, or automobile.
3. Women choose more passive methods such as drowning, poison, or pills. However, 1992 statistics reveal an increase in more violent methods.
4. Women tend to do so earlier in life than do men.
5. Married persons take their lives less often than those who are single, divorced, or widowed.
6. Incidence rises in the late spring and early summer.
7. Highest rates are among the young and old.
8. Christians have traditionally been taught that suicide is a sin: Roman Catholics are less likely to kill themselves than Protestants.
9. Jews have an even lower rate than Christians.

Why Do People Take Their Own Lives?

To my knowledge there are no exact statistics as to why people kill themselves, although there are a number of reasons why people do it. As far as I am concerned, the primary cause of suicide is to escape pain—be it emotional or physical. When the pain of life or body becomes too much for a person to bear, the escape through death becomes an attractive alternative. When the stock market crashed and the banks closed in 1929, many people jumped from buildings or used other means of taking their lives. The pain of being penniless after years of hard work was too much—out went the lights.

Emotional pain comes in many boxes: rejection by someone you love; feelings of being useless or worthless; loneliness or feelings of loss of a spouse, parent, sibling, or friend; or just feeling that life is asking more from you than you feel you can deliver. Most of these feelings are related to how we feel about ourselves—our self-concept. A good feeling of self promotes healing of emotional pain; a low feeling of self intensifies the pain. If you have a lousy opinion of yourself and you are carrying a heavy load of emotional pain or guilt, you are a candidate for suicide. If the pain can be relieved, the desire for suicide is also reduced.

Then there are some vindictive people who kill themselves to get even. Children have been known to kill themselves to get even with parents for something the child felt was terribly unjust. Lovers have killed themselves to get even with the other, often with bizarre plans to get the most mileage out of it. Some have killed themselves or allowed themselves to be killed for what they felt was a noble or worthwhile cause. The most stupid reason I ever heard was the adolescent who killed herself so that she could "experience death."

Are people who kill themselves insane? All too often I have heard someone say something like this: "Any person who commits suicide is insane, for it is impossible for a sane person to take his own life." Perhaps this line of thinking is an attempt for the thinker to pardon the victim of suicide—"Forgive them for they know not what they do."

The answer to my original question is that it is my feeling that some are and some are not insane. Insanity in itself does not necessarily promote suicide, although the persons with a valid diagnosis of insanity are out of touch with reality and in many cases are incapable of comprehending the act or its finality. However, there are some who are completely in touch with reality who have not been diagnosed as having any mental illness, neither do they show any signs of impending illness, who take their lives. They plan and carry out their own death. I can't buy that garbage of "temporary insanity" either for suicide, murder, or other violent behavior. Is one who loses control of his temper insane? If so, then anyone who flies off the handle for any reason is insane for the moment and should not be held accountable for the damage.

How Are Suicide And Disability Related?

Why all this talk about suicide? Is it important in coping with disability? It certainly is important for all persons who are involved in any way with persons with disabilities. From what I have written regarding suicide, the profile of the disabled person emerges as one with many valid reasons for suicide. It seems obvious that the person who is disabled very often has a low self image, feels worthless, has physical pain, and sees life as hopeless. Therefore, we expect the disabled person to be suicidal. When he threatens suicide there is panic. Behavior that is expected has a remarkable way of fulfilling itself.

The act of suicide can be divided into two groups: the talkers and the doers. If someone points a gun to my head and says, "I am going to blow your brains out," I will take him very seriously until I find out if he really means business. Most persons working in suicide prevention take suicidal threats equally as seriously. When one deals with potential death, either his own or mine, there is no alternative but to believe he means business until the threat is passed.

One threatens suicide and the entire community and its resources come to attention. It gets attention and it gets results. This is why the threat of suicide is the joker of manipulative behavior. It is the highest trump card in the deck of life, and a wise manipulater saves the card for just the right play. If played too often, it loses its power as high trump and becomes a bluff or a "wolf, wolf" situation. Often when the talker has abused his suicidal trump card and it no longer commands attention, he will even make a feeble attempt at suicide (one that is designed to fail) to re-establish its manipulative clout. Sometimes the designed-to-fail suicide fails to fail, and that is the end of the game.

Now I know you would like me to say that talkers are not doers, and doers are not talkers. That would make it so simple and relieve so much anxiety. Most of those whom I have known who have successfully taken their own lives made no threats—they just did it to the complete surprise of everyone. The bereaved families indicated that they had no inkling that it might happen, but in looking back most admitted that there were subtle clues they had overlooked.

One woman I knew threatened to take her life for at least ten years. She was in her thirties and confined to a nursing-home existence. She was very vocal about her desires to kill herself, especially when she did not get her way. On many occasions I was called to go out and talk with her after one of these threats. Finally I said to her what I have said to others of similar mind set: "Elaine, if you are hellbent on taking your life, there is no one in heaven or on earth who can continually prevent it. Therefore, I have one piece of advice for you. If you really want to end your life, make sure you do a good job and don't botch it." She blinked and looked at me in disbelief.

Her family, as well as the nursing-home staff, decided that this was just for manipulation and attention, and her threats were ignored. A year or so later, under relaxed surveillance, she managed to get into the janitorial chemicals and drink lye. She lived, but burned her innards from mouth to rectum. Was she serious or just trying to get attention? Did she really know the consequences of what she drank—the pain and agony in the aftermath? Was she serious and botched it? I tend to feel, with tongue in cheek, that she might have been serious, and I always keep her in mind when someone says that "talkers are not doers." The trouble is, one cannot be sure.

Many persons who have disabled loved ones live in fear that suicide is a possibility. My purpose is to temper this fear, but not remove it. However, if you *discover* a well-organized, *concealed* plan for suicide, sit up and take notice. This is the time for confrontation. Try to talk it out with the person and not be judgmental, and least of all don't come up with the how-could-you-think-of-doing-this-to-us attitude. You can almost count on a backfire from that. If you love them and need them, tell them so and why. It is astounding how much of our hurt in life stems from misinterpretations: "I thought you said," "I thought you meant," or "I thought you felt."

ARE THERE ANY ABSOLUTES?

Finally, we must conclude that there are no absolutes in suicide cause or prevention. In suicide threats we are forced to "fly by the seat of our pants"—no instruments or other guidance—just by gut feelings. Again, with tongue in cheek, I remind you to not be manipulated by the threat or destroyed by guilt if the threat is successfully carried out. No matter how we look at it, we are walking a tightrope over an open lion's den.

As mentioned earlier, in a great majority of cases, suicide is the ultimate act of selfishness, and in some cases this selfishness is masquerading as self*less*ness (I am doing those I love a favor). Often suicide is a legitimate, fleeting thought. Although I believe a person has the right to end his life voluntarily, I also believe that society—family, friends, neighbors, ministers, crisis centers—has the responsibility to do everything within its power to prevent what might have been a fleeting thought from becoming a permanent end. Keep in mind that *every* person has the emotional mechanism for suicide. No one is excluded—not even you.

Jokingly, I have advocated a single, proper method for suicide—actually a suicide kit. It would consist of 365 pills that must be taken every day for one year. If at any time a pill is not taken, whether it is number 3 or 364, or whether it is by accident or design, the program automatically cancels itself and one must buy a new kit and begin the series once again.

Seriously, I have set up programs using a calendar and two boxes of gummed stars—one gold and one red. At noon each day, after being sufficiently awake but before fatigue or pain, a star is glued to the calendar representing that day's desire—red for the desire to die, or gold for the desire to live. Using two boxes with a minimum of 100 gold stars and 100 red stars, it gives more than three months to conduct your experiment. If there are *any* gold stars on the calendar, I think you owe it to yourself to continue the program by buying more stars. If you can honestly fill up one calendar year with nothing but red stars, I will back off and say, "Okay, it is in your hands now," but I will not be able to erase from my mind the possibility of a string of gold stars that might be on next year's calendar.

My ears have heard much talk of suicide by persons with disabilities. Several have attempted suicide or had long-range plans for the act that most likely would have been carried out had it not been for a change in life's circumstances (not an improvement in the disability). There are a few severely-disabled persons whom I believe would have carried it out if it had been physically possible. In my opinion persons with a severe disability have a more valid reason for suicide than all the suicides I have known in my lifetime. However, it has only been in the last two years in which persons with disabilities whom I have personally known have taken their lives, and that the disability was the primary cause.

Much of this segment on suicide has been taken from *OUT OF THE ORDINARY*. I believe it is justified because of its importance and that many of you will not have access to the original writing.

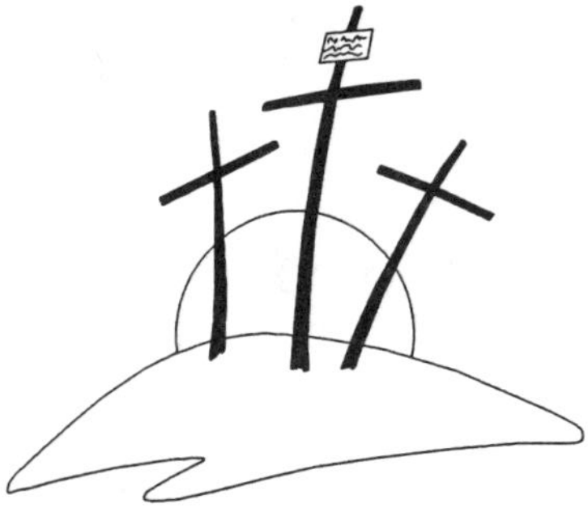

Chapter 10

RELIGION, THE TABOO SUBJECT

WHAT'S IMPORTANT ABOUT RELIGION?

God Making Comeback: Religious revival reported in world. This was the column caption in the following article in *The Arizona Republic* on 5/18/93. It brought a smirk to my face. Since when did God slip and need to make a comeback? "Chicago— Belief in God appears to be stronger now than at any other time in human history in many places in the world." It went on to state that "...everybody thought secularism would keep on undermining religion, and nothing could prevent it." Of course, as with any survey or statistical evidence, the survey had its critics, but this was done by The Associated Press, and not some religious group who had an ax to grind.

In a survey published in the Barna Report by pollster George Barna (president of Barna Research Group of Glendale, California) in 1992-93, religion was considered "very important" by 69% of the adults polled. That's a breath short of 7 out of 10 persons. Someone once said to me, "Of course you think religion is important because you are a minister." My response was this: "No, you have that backwards; I am a minister and have invested my life as such because I think it is deeply important."

If you are not interested in religion, don't bother to read this chapter, and do not complain about its presence in the book. You didn't pay for it because this book was reduced in price by gifts from those who think religion is important.

However, if your interest in religion is because you hope to effect some type of divine miracle in being made physically whole, you are in for a big disappointment. During my years as a person with a disability and in being involved with thousands of others with disabilities, there has yet to be *one* person I know who has been miraculously healed from any neurological damage. God did not intervene or change the result of the damage to my nervous system caused by the polio virus, but He did give me an attitude adjustment. God *is* in the business of making people spiritually whole no matter what condition we find our bodies!

Borrowing several paragraphs from the chapter on Spiritual Implications in *OUT OF THE ORDINARY: A Digest on Disability,* let me tell you why I think religion is important.

> "My view of man is the sum of all his parts: a physical part, an intellectual part, an emotional part, *and* a spiritual part. Because of this, I could not conscientiously ignore the spiritual implications involved in disability, and I would feel guilty in presenting what I felt to be a partial picture. If you have no interest or belief in God, this chapter is of little or no interest to you personally, but if you are in any way involved with a person coping with a disability or a family member who does have a belief or interest in God, you should be aware of how a disability can affect this spiritual quadrant and how this can affect the whole person in all phases of life.
>
> "It is my persuasion that a great majority of those who peruse these pages do have some type of belief in God. To define God in this segment, I mean that you have a belief in some non-human, spiritual super power—someone who transcends, or is greater than you. If you are Jewish, that power is Jehovah. If you are Christian, that power is Jehovah (God the Father) in partnership with Jesus Christ (God, the Son), and another member of the Godhead, the Holy Spirit. If you are Moslem, that power is Allah. Call Him what you will, for it is not my purpose at this point to try to point to my God or prove the existence of any God."

This subject was placed at the end of this book not because it was least important, but rather because it was desired that it should be the finale to our discussion about coping with disability. It is doubtful that any of you readers who know my position as an ordained clergyman would expect me to write on the subject without inserting what I feel is the prime ingredient for successful coping. To do less, I believe, would be criminal.

During the many years of counseling persons with disabilities and their families, I have seen literally thousands of persons and families in various stages of coping, some successful and some not. Was there some common thread or some thought or philosophy among the "successful" that made their coping easier or more successful?

Going back to the Barna poll, 75% of the adults polled considered the *Bible* to be God's written word and said it teaches accurately; 79% responded that the Ten Commandments are relevant today; and 76% consider sin a present reality. To me that is a mandate to continue with our discussion.

It is not possible for me to address the topic of religion from any other position than Christian. If you are seeking consolation and direction from a non-Christian position, or if you should become annoyed with the strong evangelical character of the illustrations, try to reframe them into your own religious structure.

BACK TO BASICS

As we have learned, life is a never-ending barrage of choices, some that may affect the second, the minute, the hour, the day, the week, the year, or your entire life. Some of these choices are forced by circumstance to be made in a limited amount of time. In an instance of survival it might be only a fraction of a second that determines a life-death result.

Other less dramatic circumstances we may ponder for months and years. Naturally, the choice of food or clothing for the day carries less importance than the choice of vocation or spouse. Logically, the more important decisions should be given more thorough treatment.

Our knowledge, personal tastes and values are key factors in our decision making. A small child will usually choose ten pennies rather than a quarter or a half dollar, and the frustrating experience of a youngster trying to decide how to spend his fifty cents at the candy counter is necessary experience for making wise choices later in life.

We ardently groom and school our children for making wise decisions in their adult life. Nevertheless, men often spend more time and effort deciding what car to buy than which girl to marry; and women often spend more time choosing the dress for the occasion than choosing their escort. Marriage and vocation are two of the most significant choices in life, and yet most of these turn out happenstance rather than being carefully thought out.

However, even less consideration and thought is given to eternity or eternal life. At some point in time each of us must face the question of the existence of a Creator or Supreme Being (God). Is he/she/it dead or alive? Does this Being desire a relationship with his creation, man? Is there such a thing as life after death? If there be the slightest possibility of a Creator, a relationship, and eternity for us, it would seem this should be our highest intellectual/spiritual priority to gather information, study, and make a choice to believe or not to believe.

Once the possibility of Creator/relationship/eternity has been accepted, the next step is to seek information that will aid us in our decision. The following statements are presented to you for consideration:

1) The *Bible* teaches there is eternal life. To date there is absolutely no scientific evidence or other positive proof of any kind to refute the possibility of life after death. Jesus spoke about eternity:

> *"For God so loved the world, that he gave his only begotten Son, that whosoever believeth in Him should not perish, but have everlasting life."* (John 3:16)
> *"And I give unto them eternal life; and they shall never perish, neither shall any man pluck them out of my hand...."* (John 10:22)

2) This life-after-death taught in the *Bible* is totally dependent upon the claims of a historical Jesus of Nazareth—that he actually was God who created the universe, earth, and man.

> *"In the beginning was the Word* (Christ), *and the Word* (Christ) *was with God, and the Word* (Christ) *was God. All things were made by him; and without him was not any thing made that was made.... And the Word* (Christ) *became flesh and dwelt among us...."* (John 1:1,3,&4)

3) The final test of the divine claims of Jesus Christ would be his power to return from the dead, after which He would ascend into heaven to prepare a place for us mortals to live for eternity with our Maker.

> *"No man taketh my life from me, but I lay it down of myself. I have power to lay it down and I have power to take it again."* (John 10:18)
>
> *"In my Father's house are many abiding places: if it were not so, I would have told you. I go to prepare a place for you. And if I go and prepare a place for you I will come again, and receive you unto myself; that where I am, there ye may be also."* (John 14:2-3)

Now before you reject the possibility of this "bizarre" story of eternal life and/or the claims of Christ as unrealistic or impossible, you should seek some answers or explanations for these thoughts:

1) Life is rather futile and meaningless without the possibility of eternal life. Life at its very best leaves much to be desired.

2) Buddha, Confucius, Mohammed, or other prominent religious founders neither overtly nor covertly claimed to be God, the creator of the universe. Jesus Christ did! And if he be not God, he was either a psychotic deluding himself and his disciples, or a highly effective deceptionist deceiving his closest friends, his disciples, and millions of followers for over 2,000 years.

3) To reject the biblical account of Jehovah and Jesus Christ as God creating all things, you will need a better-than-biblical explanation of man and his relationship to the universe, time, and space. The creation story in the *Bible* and in the *Torah* after 6,000 years continues to make the most sense. It sure makes more sense than believing it all just happened without divine direction in a single quadrillion-to-one chance.

4) What can be the motivating force in the change in attitude, temperament, and values that take place in many of the lives of those who choose to believe the *Bible*? When they place their earthly life as well as eternity into the hands of Jesus Christ something happens to them. Education, sophistication, and cultural differences have not changed the results of "conversion" in nearly 2,000 years.

Paul, the Apostle, prior to his conversion was angry and merciless toward the new Christian converts, stoning and dragging them off to prison. Then came the turn-around, his conversion, followed by his ministry to the gentiles, and finally his death in a Roman prison for his Christian beliefs. He wrote this to one of his second-generation converts:

> *"Whereunto I am appointed a preacher, and an apostle, and a teacher of the Gentiles. For that cause I also suffer these things: nevertheless I am not ashamed: for I know whom I have believed, and am persuaded that he* (Christ) *is able to keep that which I have committed unto him* (Paul's soul) *against that day* (death and eternity). *"* (II Timothy 1:11-12)

In stating these considerations, scriptures, and questions, there has been no attempt to be doctrinal or divisive, but to just give the framework of what has come to be called Christianity. It should be the Christian faith of a Roman Catholic, a Baptist, a Methodist, a Presbyterian, a Lutheran, any person who calls himself Christian, or a Messianic Jew. It is just simply basic biblical New Testament doctrine.

BACK TO BASICS is a backdrop for understanding and giving meaning to the following article reprinted from the Christian League Bulletin (Spring 89)

FAITH AND DISABILITY

by Robert Lovering

"This world is not my home, I'm just a passin' through," goes the short, bouncy gospel song. As we travel across the U.S.A. on the interstates, there are milepost markers to identify our location. Life also has its markers in years rather than mileposts. My memorable markers are 1928, 1946, 1949, 1954, 1965, and 1973. Each has something that to me is important attached to it—1928 birth date, 1946 polio, 1949 marriage, 1954 began ministry with Christian League, 1965 degree in psychology, 1973 move to Phoenix. Certainly we travel through our earthly life year by year just as we travel mile by mile on the highways.

As I reflect on my own life (which includes becoming disabled), and upon the lives of thousands of disabled persons who have spent time with me in counseling, there is one factor that sets some persons in an advantageous position in coping with disability. That factor is FAITH—faith that "This world is not my home, I'm just a passin' through"—faith in an eternity where God rights the wrongs of earth. It is faith in a person, Jesus Christ, to be what he said he was and to do what he said he would do. This faith can change the face of disability from life-long agony and reduce it to a short-term irritation when viewed in terms of eternity rather than this short span of earthly life.

Often in meetings, classrooms, and seminars across the country, people have questioned me about anger and bitterness in being struck down by polio at the age of eighteen, and the tough emotional and physical road back? The person without faith cannot comprehend my answer. My faith in the person and ministry of Jesus Christ ruled out anger and bitterness in becoming paralyzed by polio. After all, at age twelve my life had been dedicated to serving Christ. And just shy of my eighteenth birthday, in a Bible school chapel with Billy Graham as speaker, I gave my walking body to Jesus Christ. Four months later that body was in shambles having been racked by the polio virus. How could I be bitter or angry with life or with the Lord for messing up a body that was no longer mine? It had been given away in that chapel service.

Sure, it was a tough road back physically, but my faith spared me those severe and crippling emotional wounds associated with traumatic disability. The usual facial expressions from my audiences asking about anger and bitterness often indicated that they thought that this fellow was either lying or crazy when they heard his answer. If I am or was either lying or crazy, I have a lot of company. The difference between emotional life and death for disabled persons or others enduring a similar trauma is FAITH in Jesus Christ and eternity based upon the teaching in the *Bible*. Let me give you one outstanding story of how faith made the difference in the outlook of a severely disabled person.

My first visit with Margaret was in 1980. She was just into her forties and had spent the last eight years in a nursing home. Her husband had abandoned her when she was diagnosed as having MS. Her daughter was taken from her and placed in a foster home. Margaret told me she wanted to die. She had tried suicide on several occasions but because of weakness could not carry it to completion.

However, there was something I wanted so badly to share with her. I knew it could make a difference if allowed to penetrate her mind. From the onset I shared my FAITH with her. She was never hostile, but being an avowed agnostic it went in one ear and out the other, so it seemed.

Month by month I visited with her, and month by month we talked about God, Jesus Christ, and eternity among other subjects. Five years after that initial visit, faith became a part of her life. We prayed together and from that moment she began to grow spiritually. During this last summer, on one of our visits, she said, "You know, Bob, I no longer want to take my life. I just lie here day by day waiting for the Lord to come and get me and take me home." Ah, yes, "This world is not my home, I'm just a passin' through. My treasures are laid up somewhere beyond the blue."

What a difference this FAITH can make in adjusting and coping with a disability. I've experienced it in my own life and observed it in Margaret's life and countless others who have suffered greatly at the hands of life's circumstances. This faith cannot change the circumstances, but it certainly can change one's outlook or prospective on these circumstances. It is exciting to know that with each counseling session open to me, there is also an opportunity to share with that person or family that one thing in my life and in many other's that made the difference—our Christian faith.

* * * *

THE CRUTCH OF FAITH

Some call religion a crutch, and that it is. It is a phenomenon of comfort and guidance to get those of us who need it to make the passage through life. My wheelchair gets me through life physically; my faith gets me through life spiritually and emotionally. My wheelchair is my best friend, and so is my crutch of faith.

Let me conclude with two more stories of spiritual regeneration, again from our book, *OUT OF THE ORDINARY: A Digest on Disability*. They are in the exact words of the persons indicated.

Wayne—

"From my bout with rheumatic fever at age ten until my junior year in high school, I experienced a slowly-increasing inability to get around and had earned the nickname, Speedy, because I wasn't. This problem prompted our family physician to refer me to a specialist. He painted a grim picture: he said I had muscular dystrophy and perhaps had two to five years to live. I felt as though my life was at an end, and that an overwhelming burden had been placed upon me. My feelings of despair led me to quit school and go to work in a machine shop, but within a year my employer moved and I was out of work. I made excuses; I feared new situations; I stayed at home and built a shell around me to insulate me from reality. I was angry and resentful toward God, feeling that He had deserted me and was punishing me for some unknown and seemingly unjust reason.

One day while listening to the radio, I heard of a meeting of the Christian League for the Handicapped. I was curious and called a friend of mine, also with MD, who encouraged me to attend. My reluctance was overcome by inner compulsion, and at the meeting I was confronted by a group of people with various handicaps, but who all appeared to be happy despite their disabilities. How I envied their happiness. Up to this point I had no excuse for living. I was dead for all practical purposes, and I was only marking time until the whole ugly thing would be over. Their happiness seemed to be directly related to their love and commitment to Christ. Later I came to realize that I could know this joy if I committed the living of my life to Christ, trusting Him to meet every need. As much as I knew how, I did this.

I began to sense a peace and a new meaning to life—my attitude of despair was gone—I was certain that God had saved me, loved me, and would help me no matter what the future might hold. An evidence of that change was that the words cripple and dystrophy no longer haunted me."

Patricia—

"My trouble walking began when I was fourteen and I would often fall. My parents took me to a neurologist, who after a week of tests came up with the probable diagnosis of multiple sclerosis which was later confirmed. He suggested that I not be told the nature of my illness until later, so only my teachers knew the reason for my stumbling around. I could not understand why I wasn't able to do everything the other kids did, but never questioned anyone about it.

At graduation time I became very ill and missed the graduation exercises. I think this was the first time I realized something was seriously wrong. When I questioned my doctor his only reply was, "You have multiple sclerosis, but don't worry, you can still have children." Because this was the only explanation I received, I went to the library and looked it up. There wasn't much information, and what there was I could not understand. Also, during this period of illness I realized a need for something else, but I wasn't sure of what it was. I asked our minister to pray with me, but when we were half through the Lord's Prayer, I started to cry. He stopped and left the room rather than finishing. That was enough religion for me.

The following fall I attended business college and later went home to work in the local hospital. I became deeply depressed as I searched for the answers to all my questions about MS. Trying to do it all alone, I got to feeling sorry for myself and took an overdose of pills. The next four months were spent in a hospital being treated for an emotional breakdown. After I was discharged I returned to business college and on to a job with a group of doctors.

Up until this time I had never thought or known much about the *Bible*. I knew the Prayer Book but it seemed unrelated to my life, and the church ritual was without much meaning. A friend introduced me to her pastor who had answers—answers out of the *Bible*. Although I had not been taught the contents of the *Bible*, I had been taught that it was right. I learned from this pastor that each person must make his own decision to believe it and to make a commitment to it. I didn't make any decision, but I was greatly impressed.

Then I got sick again, but I found great, new comfort in reading the *Bible*. I had never read it before because I thought it was too difficult to understand—however, not because I had tried it. Finally I said, "Yes," to Christ and opened the door of my heart and life to Him. I had no unusual emotional experience, no feeling of sin or guilt, but just a deep satisfaction—an inner peace—of finding what I had been looking for since my high school graduation. My spiritual vacuum was filled. Now I have a new source of strength to fight off depression and to live life."

* * * *

Are these not illustrations of what Jesus Christ said?

"Behold I stand at the door (of your being) *and knock. If any man hear my voice and open the door, I will come in to him, and will sup* (visit or communicate) *with him, and he with me."* (Rev. 3:20)

"Come unto me, all you who labor and are heavy burdened, and I will give you rest. Take my yoke upon you, and learn of me; for I am gentle and humble of heart: and you will find rest for your souls, for my yoke is easy, and my burden is light." (Matt. 11:28-30)

The Apostle Paul proclaimed: *"Therefore if any man be in Christ, he is a new creature: old things are passed away; behold, all things are become new."* (2 Corinthians 5:17)

* * * *

I rest my case.

OUT OF THE ORDINARY: A DIGEST ON DISABILITY
Table of Contents

1. SETTING THE STAGE
- A. The Author
- B. The Book
- C. The Title

2. THE WORLD OF DISABILITY
- A. Getting the Feel
- B. Examining the Divisions
- C. Understanding the Designations
- D. Ranking the Disabilities

3. THE COMMON DISABILITIES
- A. Neurological Disorders
- B. Sensory Disorders
- C. Bone and Joint Disorders
- D. Amputation
- E. Heart and Circulatory Disorders
- F. Respiratory Disorders
- G. Behavioral Disorders
- H. Obesity
- I. Chemical Disorders

4. THE 4 BIG QUESTIONS
- A. Diagnosis (Doctor, what do I have?)
- B. Severity (Doctor, how bad is it?)
- C. Treatment (Doctor, what can be done?)
- D. Prognosis (When will I get well?)

5. THE EMOTIONAL STEPS TO RECOVERY
- A. Denial
- B. Fantasy
- C. Reality
- D. Depression
- E. Bitterness
- F. Acceptance
- G. Rehabilitation
- H. Adjustment

6. THE DANGER ZONES
- A. Marriage Relationships
- B. Sexual Expression
- C. Spiritual Implications
- D. Vocational Choices
- E. Disturbed Family Members

7. THE EFFECTS UPON PERSONALITY
- A. Self Image
- B. Social Development
- C. Skills
- D. Disorders

8. CRITICAL PERIODS AND DECISIONS
- A. Convalescence
- B. Retirement
- C. Return to School or Work
- D. Placement in a Care Center
- E. Suicide
- F. Divorce

9. GOALS: YESTERDAY, TODAY, AND TOMORROW
- A. Social Acceptance
- B. Architectural Barriers
- C. Transportation Barriers
- D. Sheltered Workshops
- E. Education and Training
- F. Financial Assistance

Associated Rehabilitation Counseling Specialists, Inc.

(ARCS) is an Arizona corporation not for profit. It was founded in 1974 with its mission to provide cost-free counsel to persons with disabilities and their families in face-to-face personal contact, through the printed page, or any other feasible medium.

The corporation is primarily supported by individuals and churches who feel the need for providing this counsel to persons who have been impacted by disability.

ARCS is in the book-publishing business only as a means of providing information to those who are in some way touched by disability. This includes those professionals who serve this population. All profits accruing from the sale of books are used to provide cost-free personal counsel.

Book Ordering Information

You may order copies of this book, *OUT OF THE DARKNESS: Coping with Disability*, directly from the publisher—

or

Our hard-covered book, *OUT OF THE ORDINARY: A Digest on Disability*, outlined on the previous page—

ARCS
2628 E. Cannon Drive
Phoenix, Arizona 85028
(602) 971-2867

Libraries, schools, or rehabilitation facilities may order open account on either book. Write or call for quantity discounts.

OUT OF THE DARKNESS: Coping With Disability **$7.95**
(no additional postage or handling charges)

or

OUT OF THE ORDINARY: A Digest on Disability **$14.95**
See Table of Contents on Previous Page
(no additional postage or handling charges)